SPORTS NUTRITION
HANDBOOK

EAT SMART. BE HEALTHY. GET ON TOP OF YOUR GAME.

Justyna Mizera and Krzysztof Mizera

VELO press

Boulder, Colorado

English language edition © VeloPress 2019
Dietetyka sportowa copyright © 2017 Justyna Mizera and Krzysztof Mizera
First published in Polish © Galaktyka sp. z o.o. 2017
This edition published under agreement with Galaktyka sp. z o.o.
Translated from Polish by Janusz Madej and Marta Oziembała

3002 Sterling Circle, Suite 100, Boulder, CO 80301–2338 USA

VeloPress is the leading publisher of books on endurance sports and is a division of Pocket Outdoor Media. Focused on cycling, triathlon, running, swimming, and nutrition/diet, VeloPress books help athletes achieve their goals of going faster and farther. Preview books and contact us at velopress.com.

Distributed in the United States and Canada by Ingram Publisher Services

Library of Congress Cataloging-in-Publication Data
Names: Mizera, Krzysztof, author. | Mizera, Justyna, author.
Title: Sports nutrition handbook : eat smart, be healthy, get on top of your game / Krzysztof Mizera and Justyna Mizera.
Other titles: Dietetyka sportowa. English
Description: Boulder, Colorado : VeloPress, 2019. | Translation of: Dietetyka sportowa. | Includes bibliographical references and index. |
Identifiers: LCCN 2018059838 (print) | LCCN 2018061332 (ebook) | ISBN 9781948006132 (ebook) | ISBN 9781937715977 (pbk. : alk. paper)
Subjects: LCSH: Athletes—Nutrition. | Sports—Physiological aspects. | Physical fitness—Nutritional aspects.
Classification: LCC TX361.A8 (ebook) | LCC TX361.A8 M5913 2019 (print) | DDC 613.7/11—dc23
LC record available at https://lccn.loc.gov/2018059838

This paper meets the requirements of ANSI/NISO Z39.48-1992 (Permanence of Paper).

Art direction: Vicki Hopewell
Cover design: Megan Roy
Interior design: Anita Koury and Mark Voss
Illustrations: Charlie Layton
Photography: iStock, pp. 17, 47, 71, 93, 119, 157, 179

19   20   21 / 10   9   8   7   6   5   4   3   2   1

CONTENTS

Nutrition plays a key role for athletes at every level and at every age. As an athlete advances to ever higher levels of performance, diet becomes even more important. In fact, nutrition deserves to be on equal par with training.

It is no secret that food is our "fuel" for performance; the body derives energy from what we eat. Imagine pouring cheap gas into a Porsche. The car will run, but it will not fully demonstrate the capabilities of its engine. It might even make some odd noises. If, however, we filled it with the highest-octane fuel, its performance will be completely different. It's the same with our body. We can be born with great natural talent, have ideal training and support, and have the will to train, but if we fill ourselves with a poor-quality fuel, we won't be at our best.

Diet has other benefits, too. The right nutrition is the best and easiest method of recovery for your body after training, regardless of your age, your sport, and whether you're a weekend warrior or a world champion. Other recovery techniques like massage and hot tubs or ice baths will not affect the regeneration of damaged muscles as quickly as food and hydration can because the latter are delivered directly to the blood. But despite nutrition's important role in sports, it is still neglected by many coaches, trainers, and athletes—even those at the highest level of competition.

The field of sports nutrition science is rapidly changing. But the body's biochemical and physiological processes—such as how we obtain energy from food—don't change, and they are the foundation of the craft of both dietitians and trainers. *Sports Nutrition Handbook* presents a modern approach to sports nutrition while staying rooted in the principles of physiology and biochemistry. In writing this book, we wanted to present our knowledge and the rich experience we have gained working with leading athletes in such disciplines as team sports, bodybuilding, swimming, martial arts, tennis, and endurance sports. We support all the information presented here with the latest scientific research. However, we did not want this to be another book laden with theory and the fine points of chemistry, but the most practical book for you to learn from. We want you to be able to understand the concepts of nutrition so that you can make concrete, smart choices in your training and nutrition—every day. That is why we include stories of real people whom we have encountered in our many years of work. We also give advice and suggestions that sometimes differ from common recommendations, but as you know, practice and theory are often two different things. There are many myths and unsupported theories in the world of nutrition and training, which we will try to refute based on the latest scientific research and definitive physiological and biochemical science.

We hope this book will be useful for anyone interested in sports and nutrition, especially students, athletes, trainers, dietitians, and nutrition enthusiasts.

Enjoy!

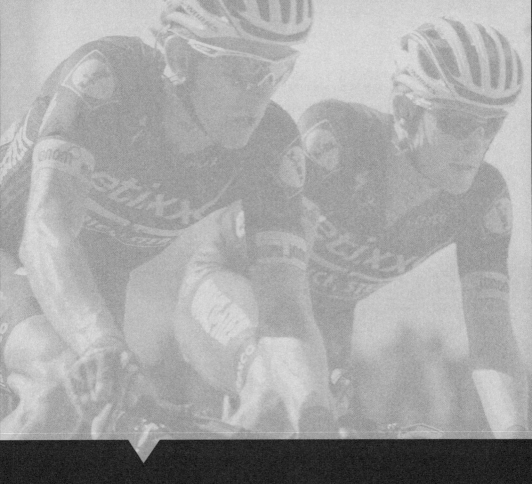

1

POWERING THE ATHLETE

Every physical effort that we make, whether it's sweeping the floor, walking up stairs, swimming, or running, requires energy. We acquire energy, measured in calories, from food, and more precisely, from four energy *substrates:*

> Carbohydrates (1 gram provides 4.1 calories)
> Fats (1 gram provides 9.1 calories)
> Proteins (1 gram provides 4.1 calories)
> Alcohol (1 gram provides 7 calories)

The body creates energy from these substrates by converting them to the chemical compound adenosine triphosphate (ATP). This process occurs in a cell's mitochondria, considered the "factories" of muscle cells.

How these substrates are used to create ATP depends on what physical activity you undertake, how long it lasts, and with what intensity. You will draw energy from different chemical processes during a 100-meter sprint compared to a wrestling match, and different processes again during a football game, triathlon, or marathon.

Our body stores only about 80–100 grams of ATP at any given moment. This amount lasts for just a few seconds of maximum intensity—when we're generating top-end power in a short time, such as a 100-meter sprint. The amount of ATP that your muscles will store is determined by your genes, so although everyone would like to have as much ATP as possible, there is no way to increase the amount available.

ATP Regeneration

We might only have 100 grams of ATP in our body at one moment, but that doesn't mean we use only 100 grams throughout the day. Over 24 hours, an average person uses as much ATP as is equal to at least 70 percent of their body mass, while someone riding a bicycle or running for three to four hours uses slightly more than that just during exercise.

To supply that much ATP throughout the day and during exercise, the body rebuilds ATP in a process called ATP resynthesis. As the body produces

ATP constantly, it needs a consistent supply of energy substrates, which come from the food you eat. Depending on the type and intensity of the effort, ATP can be created through four methods:

1. **The transfer of a high-energy phosphate group from phosphocreatine (PCr) to adenosine diphosphate (ADP), resulting in the release of ATP.** This mechanism is used primarily during short, intense efforts.
2. **Anaerobic glycolysis.** Energy is obtained from glucose in the anaerobic process during short and intense efforts, without the use of oxygen.
3. **Oxygen transformations (glycolytic and lipolytic reactions).** Carbohydrates, fat, and amino acids are combined with oxygen to produce ATP.
4. **A reaction catalyzed by the enzyme myokinase.** One ATP molecule is produced out of two ADP molecules. This process, however, provides small amounts of ATP.

All-Out Efforts Lasting Up to 10 Seconds

In very short but intense efforts, in which it is necessary to create maximum power, fuel is obtained primarily from **ATP** and **phosphocreatine** (the phosphagen system) accumulated in the muscles. These efforts spike the heart rate to 95–100 percent of its maximum. In these moments, oxygen is not necessary for the body to power the effort. In fact, some of the best sprinters run their 100-meter races without taking a breath.

When you watch runners in a 100-meter sprint, you might notice that at around 60 or 70 meters, some runners get weak, while others maintain intensity. Runners slow down because they have exhausted their stored ATP resources. They finish the race nevertheless, because the body begins to automatically draw energy from another source: phosphocreatine.

Hard Efforts Lasting 100 to 120 Seconds

While training in the gym, swimming a fast 50 meters, or performing high-intensity interval training (HIIT), an athlete is performing an anaerobic effort, but this time through **anaerobic glycolysis.** This energy system is used in efforts that bring the heart rate to 80–95 percent of maximum. This process begins when the supply of ATP and phosphocreatine is exhausted, after approximately 17–20 seconds. Muscle glycogen and glucose accumulated in the blood are converted to lactate and ATP. Anaerobic glycolysis provides energy quickly, but it is slower and less efficient than the phosphagen system used during sprints.

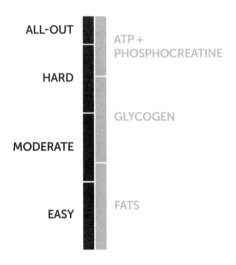

Medium Efforts Lasting Up to 20 Minutes

When an athlete performs a medium-intensity effort that lasts a few minutes (for example, running 2 miles), where the heart rate reaches 60–80 percent of its maximum, the body will begin to use ATP and phosphocreatine accumulated in the muscles. Some energy will also come from glycolysis, but at the same time, the body will look for other sources and will slowly transition from anaerobic to **aerobic processes**, where fuels are oxidized, or burned, in the mitochondria of muscle cells: Carbohydrates, fatty acids, and amino acids must be combined with oxygen (hence "oxidation") to produce ATP. This process begins after 150–200 seconds, and the longer the effort lasts, the

Table 1.1 Fats and carbohydrates fuel the body at different physical efforts

Intensity of Running (% maximum heart rate)		Contribution from Carbohydrates (%)	Contribution from Fats (%)
65–70	>	40	60
70–75	>	50	50
75–80	>	65	35
80–85	>	80	20
85–90	>	90	10
90–95	>	95	5
100	>	100	0

more these oxidative reactions become the predominant source of energy. In the next few minutes of medium-intensity effort, less lactate accumulates in the muscles because it is being burned by the oxidative processes. Table 1.1 shows the relationship between exercise intensity and which substrates the body uses as fuel.

Moderate or Easy Efforts Lasting 20 Minutes or Longer

Efforts lasting several hours include bike rides, triathlon training, and long runs. They are long, but their intensity is much lower compared to the efforts of short durations or distances. Heart rates will reach up to 60 percent of maximum (with some spikes above that threshold, of course). Here, energy derived from ATP and phosphocreatine accumulated in muscles, or generated as a result of glycolysis, is negligible. In these long efforts, the body generates most of its energy by breaking down fats—mainly from free fatty acids and glycerol.

The glycogen resources stored in the muscles still play a vital role in this kind of effort. They provide enormous amounts of energy while fats are also being burned, but when glycogen resources are exhausted, athletes are able to continue the effort thanks to the more plentiful supply of fatty acids. Because energy derived from fat is generated more slowly, athletes can become tired faster and might have to reduce their intensity. If they don't reduce their pace, once their glycogen supplies are emptied they will not be able to continue. This is the moment an athlete "hits the wall," as the phenomenon is known in running (see Chapter 2).

INTERVALS ARE ANAEROBIC EXERCISES

Because interval-based workouts are very intense, they use the anaerobic system to power the body. When athletes rest between sets, there still may not be enough time to lower their heart rate to aerobic levels.

Let's say someone is running 400-meter sprints with one minute of walking after each sprint. During the sprint, she reaches her maximum heart rate of 190 beats per minute. During the rest period, her heart rate starts to fall by an average of 40–50 beats per minute (in this case, from 190 to about 140). But what if the athlete's aerobic threshold heart rate (the highest heart rate before leaving aerobic energy production and going anaerobic) is 127 beats per minute? During that short rest, the heart rate hasn't fallen low enough to enter an aerobic state; instead, the body remains in an anaerobic phase. The runner isn't at a level of effort that would call upon oxygen to burn fat. We'll discuss how intervals do relate to fat and weight loss in the question, "Can HIIT help me burn more fat?" (p. 8).

Intervals are valuable—especially for endurance athletes doing lots of long, slow runs or bike rides—because they offer a new physical stimulus, keeping the training fresh and interesting. Such variety helps your body continue to adapt to training. In fact, adding variety to both your diet and your training is essential—whether it's for your body or your mental well-being. Interval training is also helpful because it is extremely effective in increasing body efficiency, although this is not synonymous with the reduction of body fat.

Body Fat

Fat cells (adipocytes) are naturally occurring structures in the body. Their quantity increases during the fetal period and up until puberty. After that time, the number of these cells is essentially unchanged throughout one's life span.

Because the number of fat cells eventually becomes fixed, weight gain does not actually mean a greater abundance of fat cells; instead, weight gain happens when the volume of a fat cell—and many others simultaneously—increases. It is as though you had empty balloons and began to fill them with air.

When fats from food are digested in the small intestine, lipoproteins called chylomicrons are formed, which are filled with triglycerides and cholesterol esters. Chylomicrons are eventually distributed to the capillaries located near fat and muscle tissues. Here, at an area known as the vascular endothelium, a special enzyme—lipoprotein lipase—is created. This enzyme converts triglycerides into polyunsaturated fatty acids (PUFAs) and glycerol. PUFAs and glycerol are transported to the interior of the fat cells, where the triglycerides (fats) are recreated. The adipocyte is now more full of fats and growing in size.

 How does the body burn fat?

To effectively burn fat, your body needs to be prompted to rapidly release fat from adipocytes into the bloodstream (this is called *lipolysis*) while simultaneously limiting their deposition (*lipogenesis*) into fat cells. If the PUFAs get into our organs (including muscle tissue) through blood circulation, they will be used there as a source of energy, so fat is being burned off. Fats, however, are a not direct energy source. They are a substrate that is transformed into energy after being converted to acetyl coenzyme A. So technically speaking, we don't burn fat; we burn acetyl coenzyme A. In any case, the result of this process is a reduction of body fat. And we can accelerate this process by performing physical activity—in particular, an oxygen-dependent (aerobic) level of effort where fat is oxidized.

Calories and Weight Loss: What Fuel Did Your Body Burn?

Have you ever come home after a hard, heart-pounding workout and felt really hungry? And did you not have that huge appetite after an easy workout where you stayed in an aerobic zone? It is often suggested that hard or all-out intervals will help reduce body fat. This theory assumes that by making an effort more intense, more calories are burned and thus more fat. As we've explained, it is not quite like that. Let's look at it from the perspective of where the calories come from. By doing, for example, a one-hour exercise with an intensity of 80 percent of maximum heart rate, we burn 700 calories, but fats are providing about 120 calories, while the vast majority of calories come from glycogen. However, when running at 65 percent intensity for 45 minutes, we may burn fewer calories overall, about 500, but 300 calories will come from fat (or even more, depending on genetics and the activity of oxidative enzymes). Feeling hungry after higher-intensity workouts is certainly a valid assessment, but it's the result of burning carbohydrates, not fat.

 Can HIIT help me burn more fat?

Some theories assert that high-intensity interval training (HIIT) increases metabolism after the workout and therefore helps you burn more calories during non-exercise hours. This concept, called excess post-exercise oxygen consumption (EPOC), assumes that it is not important from where we get energy during the training, but that after exercise, when we are resting, our basal metabolic rate (BMR) remains elevated. (BMR is the amount of energy utilized while resting to maintain body functions and processes. It doesn't include the calories needed to fuel physical activity.) With heightened metabolism, the theory concludes, we burn more energy at rest after intense workouts than after aerobic training.

Researchers have shown that weight training, so far quite neglected in the field of weight loss, raises BMR by 5–23 percent for roughly 24 hours after completing the exercise. However, after finishing aerobic training, BMR is also lifted, as runners of nearly any distance can attest.

EPOC happens over a period of a few and possibly several hours after training (but after several hours, the increase in metabolism is minimal). To get this effect, very intense exercise is recommended (80–90 percent of maximum heart rate); you'll usually reach this heart rate zone during intervals or HIIT workouts.

Q If I sweat a lot, does that mean I'll lose weight?

Many people complain that they exercise often, putting themselves through the ringer and finishing each workout in a puddle of sweat, but their weight doesn't budge at all. This is because they rely too heavily on the expectation that if they sweat it out, they'll surely see the pounds fall away. Remember that fat loss depends on not only the right type of exercise, but also the right intensity. The sweat-inducing workouts these exercisers undertake to no avail might encourage EPOC, but you can't use the amount of sweat as a measure of what's going on in your body.

Balanced Workouts, Balanced Diets

As you might have begun to notice, good arguments exist for all kinds of exercises and intensities being a way to burn fat. But there are differences, and we're still learning new things about weight loss and exercise.

In 2017 researchers examined the impact of low- and high-intensity exercise and HIIT on weight loss among adolescents aged 15–17. It was shown that every form of training caused a reduction in body fat, but the greatest change was seen in the group performing low-intensity training: body fat content decreased by about 9 pounds, while those who did high-intensity training lost 6 pounds of fat, and with HIIT, 5 pounds.

Regardless of which training method you choose, remember that while trying to lose weight, training is only half of the equation. The other is adequate nutrition. Only the combination of physical activity and a balanced diet will bring the results you hope for.

CASE STUDY A Volleyball Player Matches Fueling with His Training Intensity

Connor, a professional volleyball player, complained about the deterioration of his performance in training and in games, problems with concentration, and chronic fatigue. His doctors performed physiological tests on him but did not detect the reason for the decline.

When asked about his diet, he explained: "I'm an experienced athlete. I know about nutrition and have been eating healthy for years. I eat five meals daily, roughly every three hours. I eat whole-wheat bread and vegetables, and I avoid sweets." But the details of his workouts and eating patterns revealed the problem. His schedule looked like this:

Monday	>	Rest day
Tuesday	>	2 workouts
Wednesday	>	1 workout (very intense)
Thursday	>	2 workouts (including weight training)
Friday	>	1 workout
Saturday or Sunday	>	Competition

Connor ate similar meals every day. He did not take into account the fact that he trains differently each day, and therefore his caloric demand would change each day. On Monday, when he didn't train, he ate the same as on Tuesday, when he would have almost four hours of training. This meant that on Monday he consumed much more than his body needed, making him sluggish, and on Tuesday he ate too little, which is why he lacked energy in the second training session. His brain, another organ that needs appropriate nutrition, suffered from these low fuel reserves in the afternoon, too, which explained his problems with concentration.

THE FIX: Although Connor had been eating healthy meals, they were not balanced according to his energy needs. He adjusted his daily menus to properly fuel the hard days and provide less on lighter days and rest days.

RESULTS: After about two weeks of using a more balanced diet, Connor no longer felt lethargic or weak, and he stopped having problems concentrating. On the contrary, he gained an extra boost of energy and motivation, especially on the days when he had two workouts. This quickly translated into new successes for both him and his team. ■

 Why do my muscles get so sore?

The answer depends on one important factor: *when* you feel sore. Waking up with aches and pains from the previous day's workout, many attribute the soreness to lactate lingering in their muscles. In fact, this pain has little to do with lactate or what was erroneously identified as lactic acid. Instead, it stems from the following factors:

> Microinjuries, or microtears, of muscle fiber resulting from the hard effort
> Accumulated hydrogen ions
> Warmer temperatures in the muscles

This phenomenon is called delayed onset muscle soreness (DOMS) and, interestingly, it was first described in 1902 by American physician Theodore Hough. The DOMS symptoms and the microtears should resolve within one to three days.

So where—or more accurately, when—does lactate fit into the sore-muscle story? Lactate is produced by the body at all times. Even at rest, when you are not training, there is about 1 millimole per liter in your body. (Millimoles are a measure of the amount of a substance.) Its amount increases sharply when you perform anaerobic exercises. If the intensity is high (the higher intensity, the worse the effect), the level of lactate will increase rapidly until you have to stop the effort with stiff, burning, sore muscles. This is because the increasing level of lactate (usually up to 15–20 millimoles per liter) must be oxidized—broken down. In this process, hydrogen ions (H+) are produced, making the blood more acidic, which in turn becomes problematic for the body.

Lactate is formed by incomplete burning of glucose, which happens when there is too little oxygen available for energy production. After about 30 minutes of exercise, the blood will move the lactate from the muscles to the liver, where in the process of gluconeogenesis, it will be transformed into glucose. Any soreness after this short period is therefore not related to lactate because there is now much less of it in the body.

Interestingly, in 2017 some scientific studies showed that the microinjuries that cause DOMS appear to a similar extent during short and intensive HIIT interval efforts as well as during longer workouts (such as 20 minutes, with an intensity of 60 percent of maximum heart rate). Both types of training induced a mild muscular pain lasting up to 24 hours after training.

 ## How do I avoid mid-workout lactate buildup and the pain associated with it?

If anaerobic energy production builds up lactate in the muscles, then avoiding such intense efforts would prevent it. To do so, keep your effort at a controlled, lower intensity and stay below your anaerobic threshold. When you run, control your breathing (so that you can talk freely with your training partner, for example). If you feel that you are running too fast (your breath is accelerated and irregular), slow down or walk for 30–40 seconds and breathe deeply. This way, the muscles will receive more oxygen, which will enable faster oxidation of lactate. So while lactate will linger because of your previous, harder

ANAEROBIC THRESHOLD heart rates or other metrics are unique to every athlete. If you want the most accurate performance data, have it tested in a lab.

effort, thanks to the cooldown period and deep breathing, it will oxidize, remaining at a slightly elevated but innocuous level.

Another effective way to reduce the risk of acidification is the use of baking soda and beta-alanine (see more in Chapter 8, "Nutritional Supplements"), as well as drinking mineral water with a sufficiently high concentration of carbonates. Stretching is also recommended immediately after your workout; foam rolling is very helpful, too.

CASE STUDY Improper Caloric Restriction Can't Fuel an Active Body

Anna, 24, works 12-hour shifts, exercises five to six days per week, and is 40 pounds overweight. She is constantly tired, and she has noticed her skin turning more pale over time; her hair has grown dull and damaged, as well. Anna runs 6 miles three times per week on an empty stomach, performs strength training every other day, and was under the care of a specialist who had developed her diet and nutrition plan.

The goal of Anna's training and diet was to quickly reduce body fat. After eight months, her weight hadn't changed, and in fact, her fat composition increased while her muscle mass declined. She was feeling worse than before starting her exercise plan.

The most serious problem was Anna's caloric intake: Her diet was limited to 700 calories per day, while her daily demand was around 2,100 calories. The diet, with its unreasonably low caloric intake, also didn't account for changes in her activity level each day—whether she was running, doing strength training, or taking a rest day.

Anna's coach had justified the nutrition plan by believing that, with the intake consistent each day, changes in her body would be more measurable and would therefore help them monitor her progress. The coach recommended that once a week, preferably on a Sunday, Anna could forego the strict diet and eat anything she wanted, even fast food, sweets, juices, and soda. This cheat day was intended to compensate for the week of sacrifice, as he claimed that if someone is on a "healthy diet" for six days out of seven, this one day would not cause any negative consequences. Despite Anna's great commitment to diet and training, the results she hoped for never came.

THE FIX: After a detailed nutrition review and several physical tests, it turned out that Anna had hypothyroidism. The lack of this diagnosis earlier, combined with an extremely low-calorie and monotonous diet and improper training, worsened the condition and gave her no chance of improving her weight and fitness. Anna changed her diet completely: She gradually increased her caloric intake and added greater variety to the foods she chose. The more diverse diet drastically improved the supply of vitamins and macronutrients. Her training was also changed, forgoing the habit of training and running on an empty stomach.

RESULTS: After four months of using the new diet and training recommendations, Anna lost 25 pounds, and her mood, fitness, and physique improved. She discovered that her body needs a proper level of fuel and nutrition to support her active lifestyle and busy work schedule. ■

Nutrition Roundup

Aerobic efforts are a type of physical activity during which the body uses primarily oxygen. This is the case when you never get out of breath during training, when you perform low-intensity exercise (such as an easy spin on the bike). Lactate will not accumulate in excess, so you do not feel the muscle burn associated with it. An added benefit of performing these lower-intensity, aerobic efforts is that they are the most effective way of reducing body fat.

Anaerobic efforts are powered by fuels other than oxygen; you will have difficulty breathing (for example, during a sprint workout). However, this "hard effort" is a subjective feeling. For every athlete, whether they can hold a casual conversation or consider their breathing "hard" will be different. Therefore, it's best to determine your levels of intensity—via your heart rate ranges—specific to your body.

In anaerobic efforts, due to the faster breathing and lack of oxygen supply to the muscles, the amount of lactate increases. The higher the intensity, the faster the level of lactate will increase. In these efforts, you get energy from ATP, phosphocreatine, and glucose.

Anaerobic threshold is an individually determined heart rate (sometimes equated to a particular level of effort such as a specific minute-per-mile running pace), after which lactate begins to accumulate, and at the same time, less fat is burned. This threshold can be determined precisely only through fitness tests that measure the level of lactate after an athlete performs an effort essentially to exhaustion. A widely cited alternative method is to use the formula *220 – age = threshold HR* (or some variation of that calculation), but this is fraught with errors and is inaccurate. Another generic guideline that claims a heart rate of 120–130 is best for reducing body fat is also unreliable.

The anaerobic threshold depends on many factors such as age, muscle fiber composition, body composition, fitness level, and possible heart or hormonal problems. Therefore, everyone's heart rate ranges for anaerobic and aerobic exercises will be different.

ATP resynthesis (reconstruction) occurs in an anaerobic process involving phosphocreatine, glucose in blood, or muscle glycogen. To continue your effort (and to continue ATP resynthesis) for more than a few minutes, the energy must be supplied through oxidative metabolism, the components of which are mainly carbohydrates and fats.

Phosphocreatine (PCr) is a reserve fuel. The body reaches for PCr first when rebuilding ATP. It is of key importance in anaerobic efforts and together with ATP forms a phosphagen system.

Glycolysis is the process of converting glucose (glycogen) into ATP. It takes place under anaerobic conditions. It plays an important role when the ATP and phosphocreatine supplies in the muscles are exhausted—after about 20 seconds of intense effort.

Glycogen is the glucose accumulated in the muscles and liver. It is estimated that the average person stores 400–450 grams of it; about 100–110 grams is in the liver, and 300–340 grams is stored in the muscles. With low-intensity efforts, these resources can suffice for up to a two- to three-hour run, but when the run is intense, this will only be enough for about 40–50 minutes.

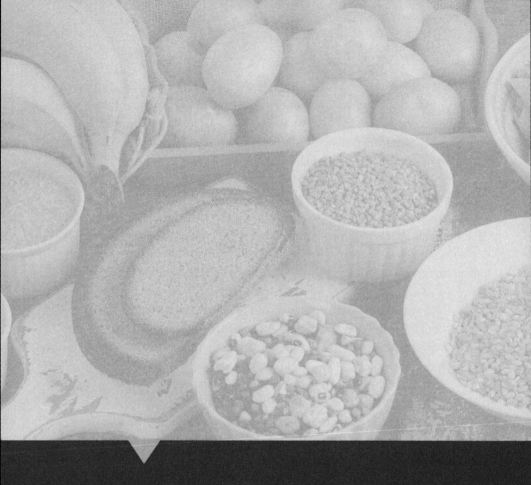

2 | CARBOHYDRATES

Carbs: adored by many, feared by some. With excessive consumption, carbs contribute to the development of obesity in both children and adults. On the other end of the spectrum, some nutrition trends urge people to eliminate carbs from their diets, which is definitely not conducive to the proper functioning of the body, especially in athletics.

So, what is the truth about carbohydrates? What are they, who needs them, and how much of them should we eat?

Carbohydrates, otherwise known as saccharides, or sugars, are organic compounds consisting of carbon, hydrogen, and oxygen. They are found in all plants, including cereals, tubers, legumes, and fruits, and also in meat. Carbohydrates are an energy source crucial to many functions in the body:

> They are the primary, cheapest, and most readily available source of energy, and they are necessary to maintain a constant body temperature, support the functioning of internal organs, and perform physical work.
> Indirectly, they help in the regrowth of muscle mass (due to the regeneration of muscle glycogen).
> Glucose is the exclusive source of energy for the brain and muscles.
> They improve the functioning of the immune system.
> They take part in the construction of cell membranes.
> They constitute a building material of structural elements in cells or biologically active substances.
> Some carbohydrates are important in regulating movement in the intestines (gastrointestinal peristalsis).

The carbohydrates contained in food usually provide 40–70 percent of all daily energy: Recommendations typically range between 50 percent and 55 percent for people who are not physically active and 55 percent or more for athletes. Some athletes (road cyclists, ultramarathon runners, and triathletes) might occasionally receive even more than 70 percent of their fuel from carbohydrates during heavy training.

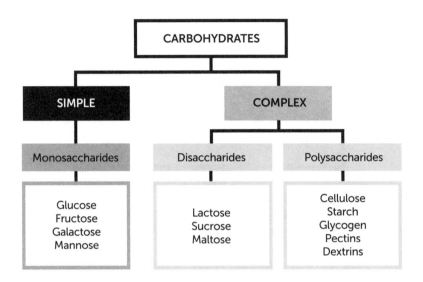

Glycogen: Power Supply for the Muscles

Glycogen plays an extremely important role in the athlete's body. As the supply of carbohydrates accumulated in the muscles and liver, glycogen is used as a source of fuel for most sports, especially those requiring medium or high intensity, such as soccer, tennis, and swimming, but also running—both short distances (except for 100-meter sprints) and long distances.

The amount of glycogen accumulated in your body depends on the nature, intensity, and duration of the exercise you do, as well as your level of fitness and the quality and quantity of the food you eat. It is estimated that we store about 400 grams of glycogen, nearly 100 grams in the liver, and the remaining 300 grams in the muscles. This amount provides 1,200 to 1,300 calories and is sufficient for 45–60 minutes of high-intensity effort or two to three hours of low-intensity exercise (for example, an easy run).

However, studies have shown that appropriate strength training and a high-carbohydrate diet can increase these values to 135 grams in the liver and 900 grams in the muscles. It should be noted that the ability of muscles

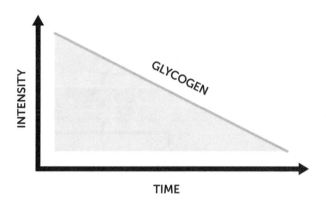

Intense efforts primarily use glycogen and burn through it quickly.
Long, easy efforts rely on it less.

to accumulate glycogen is largely genetically determined, so not everyone can accumulate such large stocks.

Type I, or "slow twitch," muscle fibers (prevalent in endurance athletes) accumulate less glycogen than the fast-twitch fibers type IIA (prominent in inactive people) and type IIX (typical in sprinters and bodybuilders). Endurance training enhances the production of mitochondria in the muscles, which are the factories where the energy source ATP is generated. So, the more mitochondria available, the faster and more efficient the reconstruction of ATP, and thus we can provide the body with more energy.

Carbohydrate Replacement After Exercise

To highlight the role of carbohydrates in powering physical activity, it might help to first consider a time when the body's fuel reserves are low: after exercise. During training, we lose significant amounts of glycogen, and it should be replaced quickly. This is particularly important when we train five to six days per week, sometimes working out three or four days in a row. When we work out on successive days, we have about 20–22 hours left to restore losses. If glycogen is not recovered at this time, then we will not be able to perform the next workout at 100 percent capacity. In the subsequent days of training, the body weakens, which in turn can lead to overtraining and injury.

Even successful, high-performance athletes who disregard appropriate nutrition are at risk of these negative effects.

Many people mistakenly think that if they eat a big, rich meal—for example, a huge sandwich—right after training, it will quickly replenish their glycogen stores. But it does not work that way. The speed at which the body can recover after an exhausting effort is limited to about 5 percent per hour. Total recovery of resources takes at least 20 hours. Research indicates that the fastest glycogen resynthesis occurs within the first few hours after exercise, especially when the athlete eats primarily carbohydrates and protein. However, this time may be longer in the case of an inappropriate pre- or post-exercise meal; glycogen recovery could even take up to 48 hours.

Glycogen restoration can be significantly improved by using carbohydrate supplements—sports drinks or energy bars, for example—as they contain ingredients that enable faster regeneration. To supplement or preserve carbohydrate supplies, you can use sports drinks during training, too. It is also very important that the first meal after a workout contain carbohydrates (and some protein), and it should be eaten within 20 to 60 minutes after the end of the exercise.

 When should I refuel, and with how many carbohydrates?

The post-workout timing of glycogen resynthesis depends not only on the rate of post-workout carbohydrate intake, but also on the quantity and type of carbs. Some experts recommend eating carbohydrates with a high glycemic index (1.2 grams per kilogram [0.55 g/lb] of body weight), dispersed across four hours from the end of the workout, at 30-minute intervals. In order to optimize the absorption of carbohydrates by muscles, the researchers explain, 55–60 percent of energy should come from carbohydrates, 25–30 percent from protein, and 15–20 percent from fat.

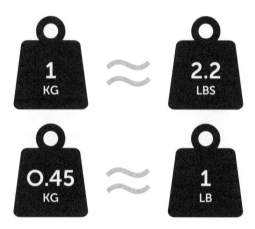

Nutrition recommendations are often based on metric units (grams, kilograms). Divide your weight in pounds by 2.2 to determine your weight in kilograms.

 Is chocolate milk a good recovery drink?

After training, an athlete needs to replenish the body's carbohydrates and protein. Because chocolate milk offers both, it has become an increasingly popular drink in sports. And the popularity is justified: A glass of low-fat milk contains 158 calories, 2.5 grams of fat, 26 grams of carbohydrates, and 8 grams of protein. (Refer to the guidelines in this chapter [p. 44] and in Chapter 3 [p. 69] to review how much of these nutrients are needed in your post-workout meals.) Research conducted on cyclists has proven that after prolonged medium-intensity exercise, chocolate milk has a better regenerative effect than commercial sports drinks laden with carbohydrates. Skim chocolate milk contains carbs and protein naturally, but they have to be added to many sports drinks—usually in the form of artificial chemical equivalents. So, through chocolate milk, you can receive a healthy dose of carbohydrates, high-quality protein to restore muscles, and basic electrolytes (calcium, potassium, sodium, and magnesium). Chocolate milk also provides vitamin B, which supports energy production, and vitamin D, which protects bones against injury.

HIGH- OR LOW-CARBOHYDRATE DIETS AND MUSCLE GLYCOGEN CONTENT

Studies have shown that in people who are on a low-carbohydrate diet (receiving less than 40 percent of their energy from carbohydrates), the amount of glycogen in the muscles after exercise not only will not return to the optimal level, but interestingly, will be further reduced during subsequent training, even if efforts were of moderate intensity. This means that these training sessions were not fully effective. On the other hand, in people who were on a high-carbohydrate diet (70 percent of the energy came from carbohydrates), the glycogen content in the muscles was regenerated throughout the day, thus increasing the effectiveness of the next workout.

The Glycemic Index: Foods Affect Blood Sugar Differently

Carbohydrates can be rated according to their score on the glycemic index (GI), a system that describes the resulting increase in blood sugar levels for two hours after the food is eaten. GI only applies to carbohydrates because fats and proteins do not cause high increases in glucose levels.

GI values are determined in the lab. A food is typically administered to several people in 50-gram doses of digestible carbohydrates. Then, for two hours, the participants' blood sugar levels are tested every 15 minutes. The same procedure is then conducted using pure glucose as a reference. The food's effect on blood sugar levels is then mathematically compared to that of the pure glucose. The resulting GI value then falls within three possible ranges:

> Low = 55 or lower
> Medium = 56–69
> High = 70 or higher

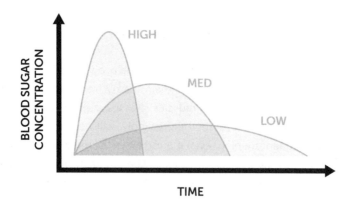

Foods with high GI values will quickly spike sugar in the bloodstream,
while low-GI foods will deliver sugar gradually.

The lower the GI, the slower the substance is converted into glucose, thus giving less energy but for a longer time (even several hours). Low-GI foods include, for example, wild rice, most vegetables, whole-grain bread, and quinoa. High-GI foods give a relatively large boost of energy in a short time. In other words, the higher the GI, the faster the blood sugar will rise, but it will also decline faster. High-GI foods include most sweets, baked or fried potatoes, cooked carrots, raisins, and white bread. (And here's a tip about bread: An effective way to lower the GI of bread is to freeze it, then defrost and toast it.) Foods with a medium GI include spelt bread, brown rice, buckwheat, basmati rice, kiwi, and whole-grain breakfast cereals.

It would be misleading to simply say that foods with high GI are unhealthy or harmful, and those with low GI are healthy. It all depends on when and for what purpose we want to eat the particular food.

In a balanced diet or when losing weight, and especially where diabetes or obesity is a concern, consume primarily products with a low GI. A moderate increase in blood glucose will not cause the jumps in insulin that have a negative effect on people of any health status. Think of what happens when you have eaten a dinner of meat, baked potatoes, and a soda. A little while later, you might be ready to take a nap. Such a high-GI meal will quickly increase the level of sugar in the blood. In response, the pancreas releases insulin to lower the blood sugar, but sometimes it decreases too rapidly. This shortage of sugar in the blood, known as hypoglycemia, gives us that low-energy, sleepy feeling.

High-GI foods are useful in the right situations, though. They're important immediately after exercise, when we want to quickly replenish the muscles' now-depleted glycogen stores. Because fuel in this moment is rapidly taken up into muscles rather than being stored as fat, post-exercise can be the best time to indulge in your favorite sugar-rich foods, such as a candy bar. Although, in reality, any high-GI food will do the trick.

CASE STUDY High-GI Foods Can Disrupt Weight-Loss Plans

Mark, an 18-year-old high school basketball player, had been trying to lose weight but with no success. He was on a low-calorie diet, but paradoxically, it had the opposite effect, causing him to gain weight at times. He felt lethargic, tired, and apathetic, and he had problems with concentration and learning in school.

The root of Mark's problem was the type of carbohydrates in his diet, not his overall caloric intake. The situation was then complicated by the development of hyperinsulinism, a condition in which more insulin than necessary is released in response to changes in blood sugar.

Mark's eating habits weren't adapted to his development, age, and training loads. His previous diets were low in calories and carbohydrates, and the carbohydrate-based foods had no variation in glycemic index. His fatigue and concentration were a direct result of not eating enough carbohydrates. And the few carbohydrates he did eat had a high glycemic index, which stimulated the release of insulin much more than those with low GI values would. In turn, this led to insulin resistance and eventually hyperinsulinism.

THE FIX: Mark could continue with a low-calorie diet to try to lose weight, but his meals needed more balance and more calories. He began to eat meals that included carbohydrates with a low or medium glycemic index, combined with more fiber and healthy fats.

RESULTS: After six months, Mark's body fat composition fell from 26 percent to 16 percent. At the same time, Mark was feeling better and had more energy and improved concentration. His nervous system was functioning better, and his strength and endurance on the basketball court increased. ∎

Glycemic Load: The Glycemic Index in Action

Glycemic load (GL) is a scoring system that lets you assess the content of carbohydrates in the food you eat. It is based on two variables: GI value and the size of a standard portion. Every food has a different carbohydrate content, and the GI is based on 50 grams of carbohydrates from that particular food. But you don't always eat that exact amount of that food, so the glycemic load can give you a better understanding of what a specific amount of food will do to your blood sugar.

For one portion of food, you can calculate GL as follows:

$$GL = C \times GI/100$$

where

    C = The amount of carbohydrates in a given portion (in grams)
    GI = Glycemic index
    GL = Glycemic load

Foods can then be rated according to these ranges:

> Low glycemic load = 10 or less
> Medium glycemic load = 11–19
> High glycemic load = 20 or more

GLYCEMIC INDEX AND LOAD OF BREAKFAST CEREALS

One of the most common breakfasts (and a snack at any time of day, in fact), cereals are often the subject of discussion about daily nutrition. So some researchers decided to look into glycemic indices and glycemic loads of popular cereals eaten with milk. They conducted a test similar to the procedure used to determine glycemic index but considered the whole meal—cereal and milk. It turned out that the bowls of cereal had either low or medium GI values. A sampling of their findings is provided below.

Cereal (with milk)		Glycemic Index	Glycemic Load
Multi Grain Cheerios	>	67.5	36.1
Cornflakes	>	54.4	27.9
Instant oatmeal	>	54.0	29.5
Rolled oats	>	42.5	23.4

As with the glycemic index, the higher the glycemic load, the faster the rise in blood sugar. Try the GL calculation in this example: 100 grams (about ¾ cup) of melon contains 9 grams of carbohydrates, and its GI is 65, so $9 \times 65/100 = 5.85$. This falls into the low GL range.

Insulin Resistance and Hyperinsulinism

Usually, consuming foods such as bread, fruit, and pasta will raise the level of sugar in the blood. Then the pancreas produces insulin proportional to the amount of glucose available. The insulin transports glucose from the blood to the liver and muscle cells, where it is stored in the form of glycogen. However, in some people, the pancreas produces too much insulin relative to glucose; this condition is called hyperinsulinism. One of the causes of hyperinsulinism is the overconsumption of foods with a high glycemic index.

Insulin resistance develops when cells do not respond to the presence of insulin; they don't absorb the glucose from blood even though the insulin is signaling them to do so. If glucose molecules remain in the bloodstream, again stimulating the pancreas to produce more insulin, hyperinsulinism develops.

Carbohydrates Before and During Exercise

The question of eating carbohydrates before and during exercise prompts a lot of discussion in the sports world. Carbohydrates (mainly with a high glycemic index) are especially important during long-term efforts (longer than 60 minutes) such as marathons or long bike rides. To reduce glycogen loss, athletes eat glucose-rich snacks such as gels, bananas, raisins, or sports drinks.

Carbohydrates let you prolong your effort by up to an hour, and for professional athletes, even longer. This was confirmed by studies on carbohydrate consumption before and during exercise. The experiment involved professional cyclists who were making a moderate-intensity effort at 70 percent VO_2max (maximum oxygen consumption) until total fatigue. At three hours before the first ride, they received 333 grams of carbohydrates (mainly maltodextrins), which resulted in lengthening the ride by 18 percent. During the second stage of the experiment, the athletes didn't have carbs before the ride but received a total of 175 grams of carbohydrates during the ride, dispersed across 20-minute time intervals. The cyclists' rides were 32 percent longer. In the third round, the cyclists took 333 grams of carbohydrates before and 175 grams while riding. In this case, their times improved by as much as 44 percent. A group receiving no carbohydrates began to weaken around 2 hours and 40 minutes; the riders receiving carbs were able to ride past this time.

Other studies have shown that in training lasting two to three hours, carbohydrate intake of 60 grams per hour (about 1.0 gram per minute) allows maximum use of energy from carbohydrates. However, well-trained endurance athletes can metabolize carbohydrates even in amounts up to 90 grams per hour (about 1.5–1.8 grams per minute), provided that they consume varied carbohydrates (e.g., 1.2 grams of glucose per minute plus 0.6 grams of fructose per minute).

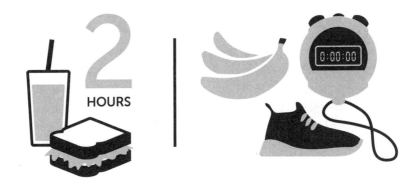

Eat a small meal two hours before a workout or a light snack immediately before.

How do I time my fueling before a workout?

You can eat a light or moderate meal about two hours before a workout to allow time for digestion. Or you can eat a light snack immediately before, provided that it doesn't bother your stomach. But be careful to avoid carbohydrates 30–45 minutes before exercise because it is likely that the increased insulin secretion will occur right at the beginning of your workout. Recall that insulin lowers blood sugar, and if the pre-exercise meal falls in this window of 30–45 minutes before, the burst of insulin could weaken the body exactly when energy is needed most.

You may wonder why eating carbohydrates directly before or during workouts can cause that spike in insulin. It's because the physical effort can inhibit insulin secretion, and muscle activity, without the presence of more insulin, increases the availability of glucose within muscle groups. Increased concentration of glucagon and other hormones during longer exercise is extremely important here. When consumed during exercise, the carbs from an energy bar, for example, will quickly get into the bloodstream and from there move directly to the muscles.

Why did I hit the wall in my marathon?

Let's explore a classic example of how intensity, time, and fueling relate. Many long-distance runners have struggled with a very unpleasant feeling that takes place anywhere between 18 and 22 miles. They call it "hitting the wall." They suddenly feel so exhausted that many of them are unable to continue at all. Why does this happen?

Runners arrive at 18 to 22 miles after approximately three hours of running at a moderate pace. This is the moment when their glycogen supply ends. Only fats are at their disposal now (not counting proteins, which are not usually used as a source of energy), but the energy produced from fat metabolism is delivered to the muscles much more slowly than the energy from carbohydrates. A runner doesn't want to slow down significantly—he wants to continue at pace or even accelerate because the finish line is just a few miles away. But, lacking sufficient fuel, the racer is unable to keep up the pace and suddenly hits the wall. This is why fueling during a long run is so important. (Recall the research conducted on cyclists who did or did not receive carbohydrates before and during their three-hour rides.)

If the runner continues his effort with the same intensity and doesn't take on more carbs, the body must use additional energy from the amino acids of muscle proteins. Then comes the increased catabolism (breakdown) of muscles—certainly not what an athlete wants or needs mid-race.

The Brain and Carbohydrates

Carbohydrates are essential in the diet also because they are practically the only fuel for the nervous system, including the brain. If you've ever skipped breakfast, did you soon find yourself dizzy or having difficulty concentrating and feeling lethargic? This is the effect of hypoglycemia. Your brain needed that breakfast to fuel up.

And the brain needs fuel throughout the day. Intense mental effort can use 90–100 calories per hour. Therefore, someone working hard mentally for eight hours can consume up as much as 800 calories, the equivalent of a solid one-hour workout. This explains why you can feel tired after intellectual work, whether you're concentrating on the job or at school, for example. The same applies when you are exposed to prolonged stress. Remember to fuel with carbohydrates throughout the whole day, especially during a period of intense mental work.

Training on an Empty Stomach

Exercising on an empty stomach, especially while trying to lose weight, is now quite trendy. Many fitness or diet coaches recommend running a few miles immediately after waking up and without consuming anything to serve as fuel. From the physiological point of view, such practices do not make much sense and can be dangerous to your health.

Let's consider this concept in someone who starts exercising to lose some extra weight. She normally eats healthy and reasonably. She has breakfast, then at 3:00 p.m. she eats a late lunch that includes some carbohydrates with a low GI. At 5:00 p.m. she starts a two-hour workout at the gym (strength training and running on a treadmill). At 8:00 p.m. she eats the last meal of the day, which is usually centered around protein (scrambled eggs or fish). From 3:00 p.m. onward, with each consecutive hour, her level of glycogen has been falling, especially as she gets rid of it almost completely during her workout. More glycogen is lost throughout the evening and during sleep, just to maintain normal body functions. In the morning, after waking up, her blood glucose level is below normal, and she's close to being hypoglycemic. Without fueling, she tries to go for a 3-mile run.

It's important to know about another concept at this point: When exercise starts, most of the blood moves from the kidneys, liver, and other organs to the legs, where it is needed more. Up to 85 percent of the blood, containing any remaining glucose, is moved from the other organs to the muscles, decreasing its flow to the brain.

So halfway through her run, she suddenly feels dizzy and needs to stop. Although the athlete had good intentions, instead of preparing for her workout and getting in some effective training, this empty-stomach run turned into a waste of an effort, with very little gain.

Some athletes can handle running low on morning fuel, but not everyone can. With more intense efforts, be careful how you prepare your body to avoid negative consequences of exercising on an empty stomach. Proper fueling will ensure you'll get the most out of a good workout.

Fueling Exclusively with Amino Acids

Some athletes intentionally don't eat before a workout but instead take amino acids as fuel. Exercising after taking amino acids can be beneficial, as many of them are glucogenic amino acids. They can change into glucose and therefore fuel the body, meanwhile protecting the nervous system and reducing the risk of hypoglycemia. This group of amino acids includes alanine, arginine, asparagine, cysteine, glycine, glutamate, histidine, methionine, proline, serine, threonine, and valine.

Eating Carbohydrates Before Going to Sleep

Many people believe that carbohydrates should be avoided in the final few hours before going to sleep, as the carbs will not be used and will instead be stored as fat. This isn't quite true; carb replenishment is essential to the performance of an athlete who trains in the evening. Remember that post-workout, muscles need carbohydrates to properly replenish glycogen in the muscles.

Imagine you work out around 7:00 p.m. and finish at 8:30 p.m. You should refuel within 20 to 60 minutes after training (in the form of a sports drink or a banana, for example). Eat another snack an hour later (depending on what time you go to bed; around 90 minutes before bedtime would be ideal). It can be a glass of chocolate milk and a sandwich consisting of two slices of wholewheat bread with a serving of sliced rotisserie chicken, for example. In total, this small meal should provide 30 grams of protein to begin muscle repair and about 60 grams of carbohydrate to restock glycogen stores.

What about the athlete in light training, in the off-season, or who is simply looking to slim down: Are before-bed carbs risky? The answer is no. While a higher protein intake serves to repair and fully protect tired muscles, carbohydrates can serve to stock the muscles for the workout ahead. Athletes planning an early morning workout, without the time or the stomach to fuel up beforehand, would be wise to snack on 30–60 grams of carbs in the hour before bed. These carbs will be fully digested and stored as muscle glycogen, effectively filling the tank for the road ahead. Post-workout, athletes looking to slim down (but not needing to fully restock muscle glycogen stores) can skip the carbs and instead aim for an intake of 15–30 grams of protein to repair and protect muscle.

By adding in carbohydrates and protein in the late hours of the day, you effectively promote muscle repair and glycogen regeneration not only right after training, but also during sleep, which often lasts seven to eight hours. If you ignore carbohydrate replenishment after an evening workout, your fuel tank will be filled up to no more than 70 percent the next day.

The amount of carbohydrates consumed at bedtime is an individual matter and depends on the intensity, type, and duration of the workout and the time between when you finish exercising and when you go to bed. If your training was short and not very intense, and your next workout is in two or three days, a full carb-reload strategy is not necessary.

Starting the Day with a Good Breakfast

You've heard it before: It's important to start your day off with a good breakfast. But opinions of what that entails seem to vary. Proponents of high-fat meals argue that fats let you feel satiated longer and provide smaller spikes in insulin levels. However, skipping carbohydrates isn't ideal. The lack of carbohydrates in breakfast may result in hypoglycemia, a lack of fuel for mental functioning, and a lack of a spark to reduce body fat (as discussed earlier, fat burns only with a contribution from carbohydrates). Breakfast without carbs also limits glycogen reconstruction, and therefore muscle regeneration is less effective. Athletes want muscle repair and muscle growth.

Advocates of a diet rich in fat claim that after such breakfasts the body tolerates much longer aerobic efforts of low and medium intensity. This may not be the case, though. In studies published in 2015, it was shown that fat-rich diets do not improve exercise capacity or training efficiency. And they directly

DIFFERENT TYPES OF CARBOHYDRATES

Research has shown that glucose, sucrose, and maltodextrins appear in fairly equal quantities among carbohydrate supplements. Maltodextrins are very common in mid-workout snacks because they are not as sweet as glucose, and the time of their absorption and metabolization is similar to that of glucose. Fructose must first be converted into glucose in the liver, which extends the time it needs to become fuel. While a combination of carbs is optimal—allowing for better digestibility and enabling the athlete to consume and utilize more energy per hour—athletes should experiment with a variety of foods such as those listed here to determine which work best for their bodies and performance:

Glucose	Sports drinks, dried fruit, energy gels, chews
Sucrose	Maple syrup, many fruits
Maltodextrin	Baked goods, cereals, rice, sports drinks

reduce the release of energy from glycogen and thus reduce the overall energy supply, limiting the production of ATP and therefore one's performance.

Supporters of breakfasts that contain mostly protein and fat suggest consuming large amounts of carbohydrates in the last meal of the day to maintain the optimal level when you wake up in the morning. However, nowhere do they indicate how many carbohydrates to eat at bedtime because the determination of this is virtually impossible. If you eat too few carbs, they will be used for partial glycogen resynthesis and other physiological processes during sleep (organ functioning, maintaining a constant body temperature, and the like) so that in the morning you may have an insufficient amount for an effective workout. If the amount is too high, it is likely that the excess carbohydrates will be deposited as a reserve in adipose tissue.

Breakfasts containing a mix of macronutrients—protein, fats, and carbohydrates—don't cause such complications, and they can provide a feeling of fullness for a long time if we balance them properly. Lastly, they will not cause a sudden burst of insulin. For a good breakfast, focus on carbohydrates with a low and medium glycemic index along with some protein and high-quality fats.

Q How many carbs do I need in one day?

Recommendations for the amount of carbohydrates (and any other energy substrate) to consume is best calculated per kilogram of body mass (we'll call it "body weight"). It's an individual matter that is influenced by genetic determinants, the degree of risk of obesity, age, type of activity, type of work performed, other health problems, and more. In the case of carbohydrates, the recommended amount per day, depending on the type of training, its purpose, intensity, duration, and the athlete's age, is usually 6–10 grams per kilogram (2.7–4.5 g/lb) of body weight on training days and about 4 grams per kilogram (1.8 g/lb) on nonworkout days.

> USE THE GUIDELINES table at the end of this chapter to find the recommended carbohydrate intake based on your weight.

There are, of course, deviations. Sometimes, especially when trying to shave a few pounds to reach a certain race weight, competitors consume 2.5–3 grams per kilogram per day on nonworkout days. On the other end of the spectrum, ultramarathon runners might reach up to 14 grams per kilogram each day during peak training. But for athletes training with an average intensity and shorter than 60 minutes, researchers suggest that 5–7 grams per kilogram of body weight per day is appropriate.

At both the recreational and competitive level, carbs play a decisive role in the endurance athlete's diet because carbs provide so much energy—especially in the first 20 minutes of effort. Muscles of endurance athletes use about 1 gram of glucose per minute of effort. In disciplines such as cycling, long-distance running, and triathlon, the amount of energy obtained from carbohydrates, especially during periods of high training load, should provide 60–70 percent of the total daily caloric value.

Carbohydrate Loading Before a Race or Competition

Carbohydrate loading, sometimes called carbohydrate charging, is a procedure aimed at increasing the glycogen level above the average level for a particular event or training period. The goal is to fuel up with as much as 120 percent of your usual stores. These resources can be increased in athletes due to the phenomenon of supercompensation.

Athletes use different methods when carbo-loading, but the most effective strategy lasts six days and is divided into two stages. The first stage is designed to deplete glycogen resources in the muscles. For two to three days, you perform a normal workout but reduce the intake of carbohydrates. If you normally eat 5–6 grams per kilogram of body weight per day, then at this stage you should lower intake to approximately 3 or even 2 grams per kilogram of body weight per day. On the third day you may feel slightly weaker and mentally fatigued, which is a consequence of hypoglycemia. But you need not worry; the amount of carbohydrates is reduced but controlled, so there is no real danger.

Now that the muscles are low on glycogen, they are ready to take up more—to supercompensate. And this is where you enter the second stage (the "loading" phase), which lasts three to four days. You can limit training, maybe doing only a light warm-up, but you replenish your muscles and consume much more carbohydrates than usual—for example, 8–11 grams per kilogram of body weight. The last 24–48 hours are especially important. During this time, muscles will surpass their original levels of glycogen and reach up to 120 percent by the seventh day. This rich supply of glycogen will not only improve your efficiency, but will also delay the onset of fatigue.

The recommendations described here are generalized. Each person is unique in his or her reactions to nutritional changes, metabolism, and genetic makeup, muscle mass, and level of activity, and may therefore need other doses of carbohydrates at particular stages. The number of days needed for a

CARBOHYDRATE LOADING IN BODYBUILDING

Carbo-loading is also used by athletes in sports that require a lot of strength and power, including bodybuilding. Why would bodybuilders need more glycogen? They perform a modified charging cycle for a completely different purpose than endurance athletes. Glycogen accumulates in the muscles, including the biceps, chest, and thighs. Carbohydrates bind water (1 gram of carbohydrates binds with 2.7–4 grams of water), so to properly digest carbohydrates, you need to drink enough water. In the last few days before a competition, bodybuilders take in large amounts of water (even a dozen or so liters). Much of it goes into the muscles, where it is bound with carbohydrates. Then, usually for 24–28 hours before the competition, the bodybuilder drinks nearly no water (sometimes only 0.5 liters per day). Large amounts of water are expelled from the body, but the water accumulated in glycogen remains; the athlete will pause training at this point, preserving much of the glycogen and the water in the muscles. When he comes out on the competition stage, he'll look as ripped as possible because most of the water in the body will be held only in the muscles, not under the skin, for example, giving the muscles a very full appearance. Water bloats the body somewhat, thereby "blurring" muscle definition, which is the last thing a bodybuilder wants on competition day.

given stage may also vary (sometimes both the first and the second stage may consist of two days so that the whole process may last four or five days, not six). It is difficult to say exactly which method is more effective. Both should be tested to check which works better for your body.

Interestingly, the Australian Institute of Sport suggests that the first stage, where the loss of glycogen happens, is actually unnecessary. Some athletes feel very uncomfortable after the first stage of carbo-loading. They feel bad even a few days later and are unable to quickly return to their best form. According to the researchers, it is recommended to only execute the second stage of the plan—the loading stage—taking 7–11 grams of carbohydrates per kilogram of body weight for one to four days, although this fourth day may have side effects for some people: Excess carbohydrates will eventually be deposited in the form of adipose tissue. (Implementing the first stage minimizes this risk.)

Regardless of the carbo-loading program, it's helpful to experiment with the process before carbo-loading for important competitions. Try a certain loading program a month before the competition to evaluate how your body reacts, the number of days needed, and the method used. This will allow you to draw conclusions and define a more precise diet strategy for the big day.

Different Types of Carbohydrates

Lactose

One particular carbohydrate presents a substantial problem for many people: lactose. It's a disaccharide (glucose plus galactose) found in dairy products. The enzyme lactase breaks it down into simple sugars in the small intestine. Insufficient activity of this enzyme causes problems with the digestion of lactose, known as lactose intolerance. Research shows that one out of every three adults has a problem with lactose digestion.

Only milk contains lactose in its original form. Both hard and soft cheeses, and fermented products such as yogurt, kefir, and buttermilk, have a much lower lactose content (basic nutritional components of a few dairy products are listed in Table 2.1). There are fairly simple solutions to dealing with lactose digestion problems if you don't want to exclude such foods entirely. Some who have a hard time with lactose can use a lactase supplement, taking it about five minutes before a meal. This often relieves discomfort associated with the digestion of lactose. Another method of overcoming digestion problems is to consistently consume fermented milk products, as research has indicated that frequent consumption of fermented milk products may encourage lactose tolerance.

TABLE 2.1 **Dairy product nutrient composition by weight**

	Water (%)	Fat (%)	Protein (%)	Lactose (%)
Cow milk, 2% fat	89	2.0	3.0	4.8
Goat milk	87	4.0	3.5	4.5
Cream, 25% fat	68	25.0	3.0	4.0
Cottage cheese, low-fat	64	18.0	14.0	2.5
Cottage cheese, full fat	35	32.0	26.0	2.0
Greek yogurt, nonfat	84	2.0	10	3.6
Plain yogurt, nonfat	85	0.2	5.7	7.7
Plain yogurt, whole fat	87	3.25	3.5	4.7

Many dairy products have a high nutritional value, and they are a very good source of easily absorbed calcium, so they are great to keep in your diet if you can handle them. Beware any myths about lactose. It in fact does not cause a blood-sugar spike, as its GI value sits in the middle of the index (46), and it does not contribute to the development of cellulite in women.

High-Fructose Corn Syrup

High-fructose corn syrup is one of the most popular and ubiquitous sweeteners because it is cheap and very efficient to make and use. It contains glucose, fructose, and a mixture of other sugars. This syrup is widely used to sweeten nonalcoholic, carbonated, and noncarbonated beverages, and we also find it in fruit juices, alcoholic beverages, and fermented milk beverages and yogurt. It is prevalent in foods loved by kids—as a sweetener in ice cream and other frozen desserts, jams, jellies, and candies.

Research shows that if high-fructose corn syrup is consumed in the first meal of the day, calories from this and subsequent meals are more likely to lead to the development of more body fat. And we process fructose into the worst kind of fat—the so-called visceral fat, which accumulates around the internal organs. High-fructose corn syrup suppresses liver function, changes metabolism to promote fat accumulation in fat cells, and blocks the secretion of leptin, a hormone that sends the signal of satiety or feeling full.

 ## Is brown sugar healthier than white sugar?

Brown sugar, although considered by many people a better and healthier alternative to white sugar, is in fact almost identical. The process of producing brown and white sugar is essentially the same, but the brown color comes from the addition of some previously removed molasses. Food manufacturers exploit the visual difference to portray brown sugar as somehow better. And many people consider it a lower-calorie alternative: 100 grams of brown sugar contains 373 calories, while white sugar contains 396 calories. Due to the smaller size of brown sugar crystals, though, there are more calories in a teaspoon of brown sugar than in a teaspoon of white sugar. The minute differences between the two sugars will not help anyone lose unwanted pounds.

Unrefined, or "raw" brown sugar is also touted as a substitute for white sugar, though. This type of sugar also owes its color to molasses, which contributes some iron, calcium, magnesium, and potassium. These minerals, however, are present only in trace amounts, and considering the relatively small amount of sugar consumed, they offer no major benefit for the diet.

Gluten

Gluten is a mixture of proteins found in some cereals such as wheat, rye, and barley, and in a smaller amount, oats. Negligible amounts of gluten can also be found in deli meats and cheese. Although gluten has no nutritional value, without it, pasta and bread would not hold their shape, and they'd be hard and have less flavor.

People with gluten intolerance can usually allow a small amount of gluten in their diet. Only celiac disease makes it an absolute necessity to eliminate all products with gluten from the menu. About 1 percent of the US population has celiac disease, and its prevalence is about the same in other countries.

Many people who want to lose some extra weight go on a gluten-free diet with hope that this will accelerate weight loss. Bear in mind that gluten itself is not fattening. Weight gain comes not from the gluten, but from other ingredients in glutenous foods: primarily sugar and fat found in foods like biscuits, cakes, and bread. It is helpful to limit these foods to lose weight.

While a gluten-free diet will help avoid the "extras" like sugars and fats that come with some gluten-heavy treats, a gluten-free diet will also reduce the supply of B vitamins, including folic acid, as well as magnesium, iron, calcium, zinc, and selenium because rye bread, whole-wheat flour, and whole-wheat pasta and cereals are rich in these nutrients.

To make gluten-free products such as bread fit for consumption, larger amounts of additives such as salt, sugar, and fat are often used, which are not healthy in excess. People affected by celiac disease should pay attention to gluten-free processed foods because they may contain less fiber but more fat than the gluten products they're replacing. Producers of gluten-free foods must heavily process wheat flour or rye flour to remove this protein.

The elimination of gluten is not an ideal solution for athletes or for people trying to lose substantial amounts of fat. If you do pursue a gluten-free diet, do it with professional guidance. You want to be certain that you're maintaining a proper intake of carbohydrates and nutrients when you remove foods with gluten from your diet.

The elimination of gluten from the diet of healthy athletes does not guarantee improvement in their sport, and the poorly executed conversion of products into gluten-free foods may even cause considerable deficiencies. Furthermore, some scientific studies have shown that discontinuation of gluten in healthy athletes does not improve bowel function nor increase efficiency.

Each person is different, of course, and it is best to test your reactions to elimination diets and then have an objective view of their effectiveness rather than be persuaded by popular and often not entirely justified opinions.

Nutrition Roundup

Glycogen is a valuable fuel for muscles in most sports, and it is crucial for medium- and high-intensity efforts such as running sprints. On average, the body holds about 400 grams of glycogen, of which 70–100 grams accumulate in the liver and about 300 grams is in the muscles. The rate of glycogen consumption depends on the intensity and duration of exercise. Proper fueling with carbs before exercise will maximize the athlete's performance.

Carbohydrates are important during and after exercise, too. Eating carbohydrates after a workout will cause faster regeneration of glycogen, so the next workout will be more effective. Consuming carbohydrates is also recommended during exercise, but their use only makes sense for long-term training (for example, sessions lasting longer than 60 minutes); carb consumption in these workouts can substantially prolong the endurance effort.

Foods with higher glycemic index (GI) values will increase the blood glucose level faster (white bread and sweetened juices have high GI values, for example). Such foods will cause a rapid burst of insulin, which can lead to weakness and fatigue (symptoms of hypoglycemia). Low-GI foods (wholegrain bread or quinoa, for example) cause a moderate, long-term increase in blood glucose. GI values only apply to carbohydrates.

Glucose is the most important fuel for the brain. If your job involves a lot of heavy concentration, or you study a lot, make sure that your brain is working at full capacity. A lack of glucose will cause problems with concentration. In turn, its excess will make you overweight, cause dental problems, and other diseases.

Do not train on an empty stomach. Although your insulin level is low after you awaken from sleep, which in theory promotes the reduction of body fat, numerous studies have shown that exercise in these conditions increases the risk of hypoglycemia. Remember that carbohydrates must be present to burn fat. Therefore, training after consuming a small amount of carbohydrates, whether in a solid form (a few bites of a banana) or liquid (a glass of juice or sports drink) will bring much better results than exercising on an empty stomach.

You can and should eat carbohydrates later in the day if you work out in the evening or late afternoon. Glycogen regeneration takes place slowly and lasts about one day (or longer if your carbohydrate levels are really low), and the most important are the first hours after training (up to six hours later). Consuming carbohydrates with a low GI value before bedtime will enhance the regeneration of glycogen, which will prepare you for your next workout. Furthermore, being fully fueled, you will be able to perform this next workout at 100 percent of your capability. If you neglect the first, crucial hours of refueling, regeneration will take significantly more time, which can cause serious problems if you are training on back-to-back days.

Recommended Carbohydrate Intake

Total daily carbohydrate consumption depends on your age, sport, and intensity of training, among other variables, but the guidelines below are a good starting point for determining the amount of carbohydrates you should eat each day. There are distinct recommendations for intake on days that you do and do not train; as energy demands change, so does your fueling.

Body Weight			Daily Carbohydrate Intake		
(pounds)	(kilograms)		Nontraining Day (grams)	Training Day (Low End) (grams)	Training Day (High End) (grams)
100	45	>	181	272	454
110	50	>	200	299	499
120	54	>	218	327	544
130	59	>	236	354	590
140	64	>	254	381	635
150	68	>	272	408	680
160	73	>	290	435	726
170	77	>	308	463	771
180	82	>	327	490	816
190	86	>	345	517	862
200	91	>	363	544	907
210	95	>	381	572	953

Continues

Continued

Body Weight			Daily Carbohydrate Intake		
(pounds)	**(kilograms)**		**Nontraining Day (grams)**	**Training Day (Low End) (grams)**	**Training Day (High End) (grams)**
220	100	>	399	599	998
230	104	>	417	626	1,043
240	109	>	435	653	1,089
250	113	>	454	680	1,134
260	118	>	472	708	1,179
270	122	>	490	735	1,225
280	127	>	508	762	1,270
290	132	>	526	789	1,315
300	136	>	544	816	1,361

Note: Nontraining day assumes 4 grams of carbohydrates per kilogram of body weight. Training days assume 6 grams (at the low end) or 10 grams (high end) per kilogram of body weight.

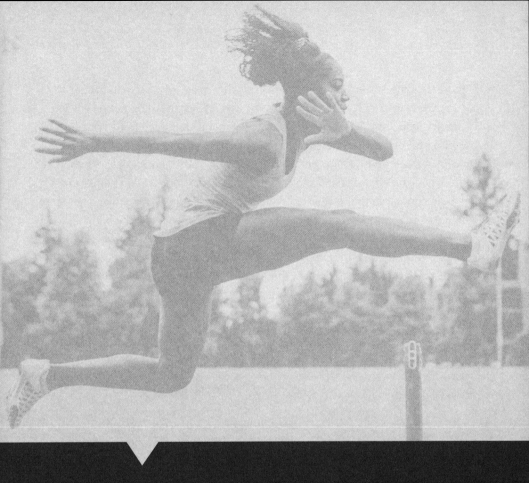

3 | PROTEIN

rotein, or more precisely, the amino acids that make up protein, is primarily a building material for the human body, especially in developmental stages of life. It is indispensable for muscle regeneration after intense physical exercise and especially strength training, where the goal is to build muscle. Protein is also important for endurance athletes, whose muscles are exposed to risks of significant damage and catabolism. In addition, protein helps regulate fluid content in the circulatory system and intra- and extracellular spaces, which ensures the maintenance of a proper balance of water in the body.

Proteins also act as transporters of other materials: They move various substances through cell membranes, and they are responsible for the transport of oxygen (via hemoglobin), metal ions (transferrin), some hormones,

TABLE 3.1 **Protein's many roles in the body**

Protein Function	Examples
Cellular growth	Development in young organisms; muscle growth
Tissue repair	Healing wounds; scar formation; muscle regeneration
Control of metabolic processes through use of enzymes	Regulation of vital processes such as blood coagulation; toxin elimination; support of immunity and defense
Regulation of vital activities through hormones	Energy management via insulin regulation
Immune system support	Antibody production
Hydration management	Water passing from the bloodstream to tissues when albumin (a protein) content in blood is lowered
Material transport	Transport of iron by transferrin; transport of vitamin A by retinol-binding protein

nutrients, and medicines. A shortage of protein in the diet can weaken intellectual performance and immune response, too. A summary of protein's uses in the body appears in Table 3.1.

For athletes, protein is especially important because it provides the body with the proper amount and balance of amino acids necessary for muscle regeneration. After you put your body through the rigors of training, you'll need protein to help your body respond and grow stronger.

An overabundance of protein in the diet is not helpful, however. In the 1970s, it was recommended that athletes eat 3–4 grams of protein for every kilogram of body weight. Today, we know that such a large amount has no impact on gains in muscle mass or faster regeneration, and it may even do harm.

Protein Building Blocks: Amino Acids

Amino acids, formed from the digestion of proteins in the gastrointestinal tract, are used for the synthesis of other proteins and tissue, hormones (melatonin, serotonin, histamine, dopamine, adrenaline, and norepinephrine),

THE NITROGEN BALANCE INDICATES PROTEIN LEVELS IN THE BODY

About 16 percent of protein mass is nitrogen. The ratio of nitrogen delivered to the body (via food) to nitrogen excreted (in urine and sweat) is called the nitrogen balance. We should aim to have this evenly balanced—at a ratio of 1 to 1. When more nitrogen is removed than consumed, the balance is negative, indicating a protein deficiency; a positive balance means protein supply is in excess. A small surplus of nitrogen is acceptable, though, because the protein will still be used for cell regeneration—for example, after intense exercise, a debilitating illness, injury, or fasting. If the balance is strongly positive, the excess protein isn't being absorbed and is removed through urine.

neurotransmitters (for example, gamma-aminobutyric acid, or GABA), as well as active peptides supporting the proper functioning of the body.

Amino acids are categorized as either essential or nonessential. **Nonessential amino acids** are those that the body can produce by itself in sufficient quantities. **Essential amino acids** are those that the body cannot create, so they must be acquired through food. The presence of an adequate amount of proteins in the diet, containing all the essential amino acids, supports not only the proper growth and development of the body, but also intellectual performance and proper immune response.

Essential Amino Acids	Nonessential Amino Acids
> Arginine (Arg)	> Alanine (Ala)
> Histidine (His)	> Asparagine (Asn)
> Isoleucine (Ile)	> Aspartic acid/aspartate (Asp)
> Leucine (Leu)	> Cysteine (Cys)
> Lysine (Lys)	> Glutamic acid/glutamate (Glu)
> Methionine (Met)	> Glutamine (Gln)
> Phenylalanine (Phe)	> Glycine (Gly)
> Threonine (Thr)	> Proline (Pro)
> Tryptophan (Trp)	> Serine (Ser)
> Valine (Val)	> Tyrosine (Tyr)

Some amino acids—such as arginine and glycine—are considered *conditionally essential.* They can be synthesized within the body from other amino acids, but with inadequate diet or other metabolism changes, their synthesis may be insufficient, so they must be replenished from food.

Although arginine and histidine are produced by the body of an adult, they are created in small quantities, and in children, they are considered essential amino acids. Histidine is important to people who want to increase their muscle mass.

In addition to the 20 mentioned, there are 4 additional but rare amino acids: selenocysteine (Sec), pyrrolysine (Pyl), hydroxylysine (Hyl), and hydroxyproline (Hyp); the latter two are found only in collagen.

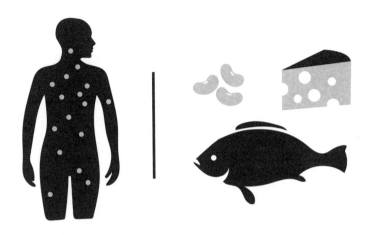

**Nonessential proteins can be made in the body.
Essential proteins must come from food.**

How the Body Digests Protein

It's helpful to understand how protein is digested because it requires a good amount of time in the gastrointestinal tract and can therefore affect how you feel during and after exercise. If you eat a bowl of cottage cheese an hour before training, for example, you may experience stomach discomfort because during exercise, up to 85 percent of your blood travels to your muscles, while only a small amount stays in your stomach and liver. With fewer resources available for digestion, the process slows down, and it can give you a full or even painful feeling in your stomach.

Digestion of proteins begins in the stomach, where there is a highly acidic environment. Here, pepsin is secreted to begin the process. After this early digestive step, the nutrients move to the duodenum, where pancreatic secretions containing enzymes further digest the proteins. The digested proteins are divided into shorter segments, or peptides, and the enzymes here release a few amino acids. Next, the proteins are moved to the small intestine, where the exopeptidase enzymes begin to act. The digested proteins stimulate the formation of dipeptides and amino acids. This form of protein is taken to the liver. Then the amino acids are transported to all tissues so that the cells can conduct protein synthesis.

The breakdown and synthesis of amino acids occur in the body constantly, and the speed of this process is determined by both the source of protein and what's going on in the body (see Table 3.2). Hunger causes faster breakdown of proteins in the liver, and when protein synthesis activity in the muscles increases, protein digestion in the gut slows.

 How much protein should I eat?

The amount of protein an athlete needs can be determined in a few different ways. As a percentage of total calorie consumption, protein should represent 13–16 percent of the daily calorie intake. For example, if a powerlifter consumes 4,000 calories per day, 520–640 calories should come from proteins. In Chapter 1, we noted that 1 gram of protein contains 4.1 calories. So a provision of 520 calories from proteins would equate to about 127 grams of protein.

USE THE GUIDELINES table at the end of this chapter to find the recommended protein intake based on your weight.

For a more accurate calculation of your protein requirements, it's helpful to use a formula based on body weight. The average person who is fairly inactive (not an athlete or even an avid exerciser) requires an intake of at least 0.8 grams of protein per kilogram (0.36 g/lb) of body weight per day. This protein should come from a variety of sources in order to ensure adequate intake of all essential amino acids.

The situation is different for athletes. It is estimated that the athlete's average demand is 80–100 percent higher than that of a healthy sedentary person, in fact. This is because the body needs more protein to adapt to training, enabling the development of muscle mass, strength, and endurance.

The amount of protein you should consume is a very individual matter. It's necessary to consider not only your sport, but also your fitness level (whether

TABLE 3.2 The body needs time to digest proteins

Type of Protein		Digestion Time
Fat-free milk or cottage cheese	>	About 1.5 hr.
Cottage cheese	>	2 hr.
Hard cheese	>	4–5 hr.
Boiled egg	>	45 min.
Lean fish (cod)	>	30 min.
Fatty fish (salmon)	>	45–60 min.
Chicken (skinless)	>	1.5–2.0 hr.
Turkey (skinless)	>	2.0–2.5 hr.
Beef	>	2.5 hr.
Pork	>	4.5–5.0 hr.

Note: Digestion times apply to people with no digestive problems.

you are an amateur or professional, for example), the amount or intensity of training each week, where you are in a training period (preparation, buildup, or peak, for example), your metabolic rate, food intolerances, and weight concerns. According to the recommendations of the Academy of Nutrition and Dietetics (formerly the American Dietetic Association) and the American College of Sports Medicine, dietary protein intake necessary to support metabolic adaptation, repair, regeneration, and protein turnover generally ranges from 1.2 to 2.0 grams of protein per kilogram of body weight per day (0.55–0.90 g/lb). Higher intakes are needed during times of heavy training or when limiting overall calorie intake.

These are general recommendations. More detailed information for specific sports can be found in Chapter 6, "Sample Meal Plans." Table 3.3 lists the overall protein content, which differs from quality, of some common foods.

It is estimated that the body of an average healthy adult male exchanges around 140 grams (about 5 ounces) of protein throughout the day. Proteins perform various functions, and eventually they wear out and have to be replaced. During physical exertion, the same amount of new protein is created as is worn out. This protein exchange is measured by the nitrogen balance. As mentioned earlier, the nitrogen balance should be preserved at 1 to 1 (some exceptions for certain sports are discussed in Chapter 6, "Sample Meal Plans").

We do not need to *consume* 5 ounces of protein per day to maintain the nitrogen balance, however. Half of this amount is accounted for by protein being recycled. The body's own nonessential proteins are used up and then rebuilt. The other half of the total protein needed is provided through food.

TABLE 3.3 **Protein content in selected foods**

Food	Protein Content (grams per 100 grams of food)
Lentils	25
Sunflower seeds	24
Turkey	21–24
Chickpeas	20
Chicken	19–23
Beef	18–21
Pork	15–19
Fish	8–19
Cottage cheese	12
Tofu	12
Egg whites	11

Note: Protein content will vary depending on particular variety of a given product or manufacturer. Values shown are for general reference.

CASE STUDY A Bodybuilder's High-Protein Diet Goes a Little Too Far

Tom, 27, is an amateur bodybuilder. He complained about chronic constipation, colic, and a frequently bloated stomach. This condition had lasted for seven months, marked by discomfort, especially in his gut, and a persistent ill feeling.

At the urging of his colleagues at the gym, Tom had been eating a high-protein diet, which is common in bodybuilding sports. He consumed 3–4 grams of protein per kilogram of body weight per day. For his weight of 82 kilograms (181 lb), that meant 246–328 grams of protein. He would often eat rice with chicken and very few servings of fruits and vegetables. His fiber intake was therefore too low, which caused trouble in the intestines and the ability to have comfortable bowel movements.

Excess protein in the diet is harmful: It acidifies the body and causes intestinal problems, which can manifest as a bloated belly and constipation. In addition, when the intestines are not functioning properly, the absorption of other energy substrates, vitamins, and minerals deteriorates, further disturbing the body balance.

THE FIX: Tom reduced his protein intake to less than 2 grams per kilogram of body weight per day, which is still a sufficient amount to build muscle mass. In addition, he added more healthy fats and suitable amounts of carbohydrates with a higher share of vegetables, which provided more fiber (about 40 grams of fiber per day). For the fiber to do its job (improving bowel movements), an appropriate amount of fluids is necessary, too. So Tom was advised to drink about 1 gallon of water per day (water intake can be based on an athlete's body weight and the intensity and duration of their workouts).

RESULTS: After eight weeks of this diet, Tom no longer had problems with constipation, and his stomach wasn't bloated and hard. His overall well-being and progress in training also improved. ■

Protein Absorption and Biological Value

Whether from plants or animals, proteins vary in how much can actually be absorbed into the body. This *bioavailability* depends on the amino acid profile of a food as well as other nutritional components. The more protein the body can digest and absorb from a food, the higher quality it's considered to have.

A scoring system of biological value (BV) is sometimes used to rate protein bioavailability. The BV is a reflection of the percentage of the protein that can be absorbed in the body, becoming part of the daily quantity of essential protein. Recall that the body needs on average 70 grams of protein through food (out of 140 grams of protein in use each day). And athletes need more, in fact. A food can only provide a certain percentage (its BV) of its total protein. So a chicken breast containing 20 grams of protein, while highly bioavailable, would likely still provide slightly less than 20 grams to the body. In general, animal protein sources and especially dairy are highly biologically available to the body, whereas plant sources are more limited (see Table 3.4). For example, to get the necessary 70 g of protein from peas, you need to eat as much as 116 grams, because their BV can be as low as about 60.

Remember, however, that the body has a limited capacity when it comes to how much protein it can digest and use in one sitting, making it important to spread your protein intake across several meals or throughout the day.

 Does animal protein cause bones to lose minerals?

For a few decades, it was believed that animal protein reduces bone mineral content and that vegetable protein increases calcium absorption. But our understanding is changing with new findings. One study in postmenopausal women showed that when meat protein was replaced with soy protein, the women did not retain any more calcium. There are no reliable arguments confirming the superiority of vegetable protein over animal protein in their impact on calcium metabolism, the risk of bone fractures, or the incidence of osteoporosis.

TABLE 3.4 Biological values of foods indicate how much protein can be absorbed

Food	Biological Value (BV)
Eggs	95–100
Whey protein	95
Milk	85
Fish	80–85
Pork	80
Casein supplement	80
Poultry	77
Cheese	71
Beef	70–75
Soybeans	64–80
Beans	62–68
Peas	48–69
Lentils	41–58

Note: Greater bioavailability is indicated by higher numbers on a scale of 1 to 100.

High-Protein Diets

High-protein diets have long been suggested as an effective plan for losing weight. In essence, they advise people to eat more protein and minimize carbohydrates and fats. But this is not the healthiest approach: You may lose weight, but with a risk of side effects and complications.

High-protein diets take advantage of postprandial thermogenesis. It is a process that intensifies during digestion, absorption, processing, and storage of food and lasts for several hours after eating a meal. Thermogenesis is, simply put, increased heat production. This process is directly related to increased energy consumption and thus the use of more calories. We experience this

OTHER METHODS OF DETERMINING THE QUALITY OF PROTEIN

The protein digestibility-corrected amino acid score (PDCAAS), a rating from 0 to 1, denotes higher-quality proteins with higher values. Studies have confirmed that the amino acid composition of egg whites (ovalbumin) and milk proteins are the closest to the composition of proteins in the human body, so they are used as a reference point (with a value of 1) to compare the nutritional value of other proteins in the diet. Among plant foods, soy protein has the highest quality. Producers of protein supplements use this rating to determine which proteins to use as ingredients.

The protein efficiency ratio (PER), though not used as often anymore, rates foods by calculating the body weight gain (of laboratory test animals) in grams per each gram of protein consumed. The following table shows the PDCAAS and PER ratings for some common protein-based foods.

Food	Protein Digestibility-Corrected Amino Acid Score (PDCAAS)	Protein Efficiency Ratio (PER)
Egg	1.0	3.4
Milk	1.0	3.1
Casein supplement	1.0	2.9
Whey supplement	1.0	3.4
Beef	0.92	2.1–2.5
Soybeans	0.91	1.3–2.3
Peas	0.73	1.0–1.5
Lentils	0.52	0.6–1.1

mechanism after each meal, but the greatest thermogenesis occurs after the consumption of protein. Studies have shown that protein increases metabolism by up to 25 percent. High-protein diets therefore accelerate the reduction of body fat, but mainly when we also stop consuming carbohydrates or limit them as much as possible. Unfortunately, in most cases, people who forgo carbohydrates are unable to maintain such a diet for longer than a few weeks. They may lose several pounds, but after a while, most of them return to their old habits of eating more carbohydrates.

High-protein diets used for weight loss can lack the nutritional diversity offered by more balanced plans, whose variety comes from the presence of fruits, grains, and vegetables in addition to the protein sources. In high-protein diets, there can be a noted absence of nutrients such as healthy fats, which support the endocrine system and cell membrane construction, and electrolytes such as potassium (supporting the heart), magnesium (regulating the nervous system), and sodium (responsible for fluid management). Eliminating these ingredients from the diet may therefore result in a number of side effects, manifesting as lack of concentration, irritability, weakness, and even fainting. A healthier solution for weight loss is a properly balanced diet combined with appropriate physical activity done three to four times per week.

Excess Protein in Strength Sports

It is often thought that increased protein intake, especially for athletes in strength sports or the martial arts, will bring about a rapid increase in strength and muscle mass. Research has confirmed that intensive strength training (not to mention overtraining), performed often enough, overloads the body, stimulating catabolic processes and the breakdown of body protein. To prevent these problems, bodybuilders or weight lifters, for example, would eat large amounts of protein. However, although in this situation the protein is an essential substrate that should not be scarce, its excess will not offer any benefits. The unused protein will be transformed in the liver into urea, which will be excreted with the urine.

KIDNEY HEALTH DEPENDS ON APPROPRIATE PROTEIN CONSUMPTION

Evidence of how high protein levels affect the body is found in the kidneys. Research has shown that eating more protein than the body needs can cause intense protein decomposition, which increases the amount of nitrogen compounds and, as a result, additional load on the kidneys and liver. Some metabolic problems can arise, including excessive acidification and even certain diseases. This happens mainly in the case of long-term protein overconsumption, often for several years.

In people with renal insufficiency—poorly functioning kidneys—restricting protein is essential for their treatment. A diet with even moderate levels of protein works unfavorably because the waste products urea and creatinine form in higher quantities. These compounds are not excreted by inefficient kidneys and gradually accumulate in the body, leading to an overload of toxins. People with renal insufficiency should eat 0.6–0.8 grams of protein per kilogram of body weight per day (35–55 grams per day). In extreme cases, the protein limits may be even more strict (0.3–0.6 grams per kilogram of body weight per day).

The liver and kidneys are the most important organs that neutralize and excrete toxins from the body. However, they have limited capacity to remove uric acid, which is a metabolite of protein. Within 24 hours, these organs are able to remove about 8 grams of uric acid, while consumption of 500 grams (1.1 lb) of meat causes the formation of 18 grams of uric acid. Therefore, some of the acid remains in the body in the form of deposits and in the long run leads to diseases such as gout, rheumatism, and arthritis. Excessive amounts of acidic compounds in the blood also cause the kidney cells to lose citrates, which are needed to neutralize acids and are involved in energy production. Through citrate deficiency come problems including kidney stones, and it leads to a vicious cycle: The more acids in the body, the weaker the kidneys, and the weaker the kidneys, the more acids in the body.

As advocated by some researchers, the minimum amount of protein necessary to optimize muscle regeneration in strength-sport athletes should be about 0.8 grams per kilograms of body weight per day, although for professionals, higher amounts are recommended: up to 1.5–1.7 grams per kilogram of body weight per day.

Studies have shown that increasing protein intake from 1.35 grams to 2.62 grams per kilogram of body weight per day did not lead to an increase in strength and muscle mass in men (aged about 22 years) practicing strength-based sports. But recently, other studies have shown that short-term use of a high-protein diet (2.8 grams per kilogram of body weight per day) may have a beneficial effect on improving well-being by reducing stress and fatigue. However, these higher quantities should not be used for longer than about two weeks.

Consuming too much protein for a long time (even up to 4–5 grams per kilogram of body weight per day), which applies to bodybuilders, among others, isn't recommended. After all, the body has a limited capacity to absorb protein, and such huge quantities are not fully absorbed, even when using supplements to aid protein development. And although any excessive amount of protein is not fully absorbed, it's not benign, either, because the body must process the excess protein to remove it.

 Can eating too much protein cause gout?

Gout is a long-term metabolic disease involving pain in joints due to increased levels of uric acid in the blood and the deposition of urate salts in tissues and joints. Uric acid is the final by-product of purines, which are found in many foods. The majority of people who develop gout are men 30–50 years old. Studies have shown that one of the factors causing gout is the consumption of excessive amounts of protein, which can stress the kidneys and subsequently cause the rise in uric acid that leads to the urate salt depositions.

As explained earlier, the body can become more acidic when protein is consumed in large quantities. However, at recommended amounts, protein can actually reduce acidic conditions in the body. This is because the protein-forming amino acids are amphoteric compounds, meaning they can behave like an acid or a base.

The acidic or acidifying amino acids include aspartic and glutamic acids as well as sulfuric amino acids, which are found in meat. The basic (deacidifying) amino acids include lysine, arginine, histidine, and beta-alanine.

Animal Sources of Protein

We have already mentioned that although the amount of protein in the diet is important, the particular variety of amino acids is also critical. Proteins most similar to those in the human body, found in chicken eggs and milk, are considered optimal.

Consider the findings of a study that followed the development and diets of children in rural Kenya over two years. The children who received animal proteins in their diet developed faster both physically and intellectually than those remaining on a vegetarian diet.

The composition of different protein sources affects the functioning of the nervous system and the intellectual performance of the brain. All the amino acids necessary for their proper development and functioning are present in egg, meat, milk, and fish proteins. A complete protein, rich in sulfuric amino acids, ensures greater brain uptake of not only tryptophan but also branched-chain amino acids, improving concentration, reflexes, and alertness.

The peptides formed from milk proteins are important for the functioning of the brain. These include endorphins, enkephalins, and dynorphins, neurotransmitters with an opioid effect (similar to that of morphine or codeine), which stimulate the activity of the central nervous system in adults but can cause drowsiness in small children.

Dairy Products and Calcium

Dairy products are one of the best sources of calcium per typical serving size (see Table 3.5). Calcium from milk can be supplemented with whole-grain cereal products, vegetables, and legumes, but these foods contain smaller amounts, and calcium absorption is limited by the presence of caffeine, phytic acid (in wheat bran), oxalic acid (in spinach and rhubarb), insoluble fiber, and high fat or phosphorus content.

The amount of calcium absorbed from a food varies from 10 percent to 40 percent. It depends on how soluble the particular form of calcium is and the composition of the athlete's overall diet. About 32 percent of calcium is absorbed from milk and dairy products. Getting the most out of calcium depends on the presence of another element: phosphorus. If the intake of phosphorus becomes excessive, the parathyroid hormone (PTH) will be secreted

TABLE 3.5 **Calcium is provided by a variety of foods**

Food		Calcium Content (milligrams per 100 grams of food)
Poppy seeds	>	1,400
Cheese	>	390–1,380
Almonds	>	239
Soybeans	>	197
Dried figs	>	160
Yogurt	>	130–170
Milk	>	110–120
Buttermilk	>	110
Kefir	>	103
Egg, whole	>	50
Broccoli	>	48

at higher levels, which can exacerbate osteoporosis. This problem most often occurs in athletic women, in whom the demand for calcium increases significantly, up to 2,000 milligrams per day. In comparison, the less active woman needs around 1,200 milligrams of calcium per day.

The quantities in Table 3.5 point to an important consideration about serving size and nutrient intake. Although almonds or poppy seeds contain more calcium per gram, note that the quantity of calcium shown is based on 100 grams of each food. It is probably easier to eat 0.8 cup (250 g) of yogurt than 1 cup (100 g) of almonds to get the same amount of calcium, so you'll likely get more calcium from a meal with yogurt than one with a reasonable serving of almonds. And in balancing serving size and calcium content, you should also take into account the food's caloric offering.

Antibiotics in Meat

For those athletes who do eat meat, it's important to eat high-quality meats, particularly those certified to have never been treated with antibiotics. Meats that are USDA certified as organic fall into this category and are often the easiest to find.

The use of antibiotics in animals and humans accelerates the development of bacterial resistance to antibiotics and disinfectants. Bacterial enzymes that can inactivate antibiotics have also become more prominent. With the abundance of antibiotic treatments, both animals and humans have suffered a rise in infections from pathogenic fungi, viruses, and other diseases, too.

When we remove antibiotics from the food sources we raise, grow, and eat, the bacterial population's ability to resist antibiotics decreases, as do the unintended side effects. Whenever possible, it's best to buy meat from safe and trusted sources who can verify the meat has never been treated with antibiotics.

The Simple Egg

As eggs offer high-quality protein and are widely available and easy to prepare, they can be a great part of an athlete's nutrition plan.

Q Are raw eggs okay to eat, and are they good for you?

Raw eggs contain the protein avidin, which reduces the body's levels of biotin (vitamin H, the deficiency of which can cause muscle pain and intestinal and skin problems). Consumed in excess, raw egg whites can lead to biotin deficiency. It is best to at least lightly cook the egg so that the avidin is denatured, becoming harmless to biotin. Other proposed reasons for eating raw eggs—retaining more vitamins and optimizing muscle gains—are unsubstantiated, so it might be best to cook them for the sake of biotin and food safety.

Eggs Provide Important Vitamins and Nutrients

People who cannot eat dairy products, which are a common source of calcium, can take advantage of egg shells. The calcium compounds that support the shell are very easily absorbed by the human body (a bioavailability of almost 90 percent compared to 30 percent in dairy products). If the idea of cooking and eating an egg shell sounds odd to you, look for egg shells in powder form, which you can add to other foods as you prepare them, such as a smoothie.

Eggs have one more valuable element, the membrane, which is a source of highly absorbable collagen. The membranes have a beneficial effect on joints and tendons not only because of collagen, but also because of the presence of chondroitin, glucosamine, and hyaluronic acid, which are some of the essential elements of connective tissue. According to some studies, after eight weeks of a diet supplemented with these membrane components, joint pain and stiffness are relieved and joint functionality can be improved.

Eggs Don't Only Come from Chickens

Hen eggs aren't the only eggs offering high-quality proteins. Quail eggs can be an alternative for people with chicken egg allergies. Their flavor is similar to chicken eggs, and they contain more minerals (iron, calcium, phosphorus) and vitamin B2. Three quail eggs equate to about one chicken egg.

Most people cook eggs either in a frying pan, by poaching or hard-boiling them, or sometimes, in a microwave. The outcomes are different, but the nutritional benefits of the egg don't change significantly. Scientific research does not support the theory that microwave ovens negatively affect the quality of proteins. The heat will change their volume due to denaturation, but it does not significantly change their nutritional value.

Because eggs solidify at 140°F, which is lower than the temperature point where butter starts to burn and form the toxin acrolein, it is safe to cook eggs with butter, unlike other foods that require higher cooking temperatures. The nutrients in soft-boiled eggs, cooked for up to 4 minutes, are best absorbed. Boiling eggs for too long (more than 10 minutes) results in loss of vitamins and a drop in the nutritional value of the protein by up to 40 percent. In addition, it leads to sulfur reacting with iron, causing the green lining around the egg yolk. So regardless of cooking method, it may be best to avoid long cook times and high heat so that you get the most out of the egg.

Plant Sources of Protein

Vegetable proteins are very important in the diet. However, while these can cover the demand for protein of sedentary people, for athletes (especially at higher levels of competition), it is not usually feasible to fully replace high-value animal proteins with vegetable proteins.

Due to the low content of lysine, methionine, valine, and leucine, most plants are a source of small amounts (1–2 percent) of protein, and they offer a lower nutritional value. But some plants do offer a much higher protein content (21–25 percent), such as soybeans, peas, lentils, and beans. Soy has a very high nutritional value but is still lower than complete animal protein. In particular, soy differs in the amount of amino acids containing sulfur. And it contains numerous chemicals undesirable for proper nutrition, such as phytic acid, tannins, and gas-forming compounds. There is also some evidence that soy contains excessive amounts of inexpedient phytoestrogens that increase the risk of cancer (although in some populations, they have a protective effect).

Plant products do not contain creatine, which is present in meat. While the body is able to make creatine from other amino acids, during intense physical efforts it may not be able to cover its demand for this compound. Therefore, providing it via food can help maintain appropriate levels.

Many people overlook the proteins available in vegetables, grains, legumes, and supplements and may not even count them in their tally of daily protein intake, claiming that they are incomplete and therefore irrelevant. Although plant proteins don't always provide a supply of all amino acids, they provide most of them, so they shouldn't be completely disregarded.

Nutrition Roundup

Protein is used primarily as building material for the body, and it also supports the body's metabolism and immune system. It takes part in post-workout regeneration, is especially important in the diet of children and adolescents, not only when they are training, but also for their growth, when they have an increased demand for proteins. Protein is made of amino acids. Some of them can be produced by our body, but we must acquire some types of amino acids through diet.

Athletes should consume 1.2–2 grams of protein per kilogram (0.55–0.90 g/lb) of body weight per day. The amount of protein needed depends on the athlete's sport, phase of training, performance level, and frequency and intensity of training. Excess protein is not absorbed by the body, and it can be harmful, so eating too much protein is not justified. Protein demand in non-athletes can be about 0.8–1 gram of protein per kilogram (0.36–0.45 g/lb) of body weight per day.

Vegetable protein cannot entirely replace complete animal protein, which provides all of the amino acids needed for normal development of children and adolescents, supports immune processes, and is also necessary for the brain—improving concentration, reflexes, and alertness. For athletes, especially professionals, animal protein seems necessary to support the body to maintain optimal performance. Plant protein should be included as 50 percent of the total daily intake.

Recommended Protein Intake

Daily recommended quantities of protein depend on your level of activity, age, sex, and muscle-growth goals, among other factors. Ranges shown in these guidelines are for endurance athletes; intake can be slightly higher for strength sports.

Body Weight			Daily Protein Intake	
(pounds)	**(kilograms)**		**Low End (grams)**	**High End (grams)**
100	45	>	54	91
110	50	>	60	100
120	54	>	65	109
130	59	>	71	118
140	64	>	76	127
150	68	>	82	136
160	73	>	87	145
170	77	>	93	154
180	82	>	98	163
190	86	>	103	172
200	91	>	109	181
210	95	>	114	191
220	100	>	120	200

Continues

Continued

Body Weight			Daily Protein Intake	
(pounds)	**(kilograms)**		**Low End (grams)**	**High End (grams)**
230	104	>	125	209
240	109	>	131	218
250	113	>	136	227
260	118	>	142	236
270	122	>	147	245
280	127	>	152	254
290	132	>	158	263
300	136	>	163	272

*Note: Recommended protein intake ranges from 1.2 grams
(low end) to 2.0 grams (high end) per kilogram of body weight.*

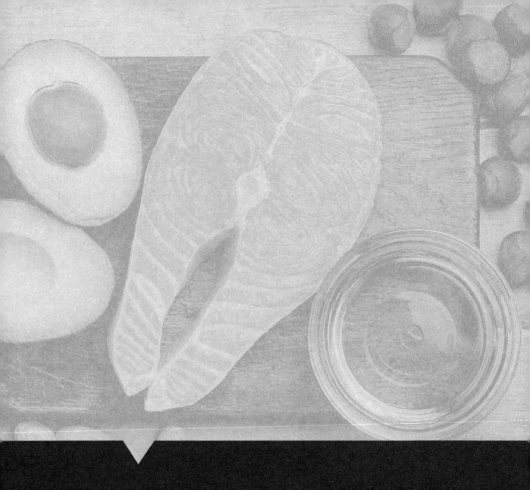

4 FATS

Fats are essential to life and should be a regular part of the diet. Fats, or lipids, are often given a bad name, but they perform several functions that support a healthy body:

> Fats are essential elements of cell membranes.
> Fats surround the internal organs, including the heart, kidneys, and liver.
> Fats have an active role in the transport of vitamins A, D, E, and K, and they also significantly affect the hormonal balance, which is especially important for people as they mature—and also for athletes.
> Fats cover and protect nerve cells in structures called myelin sheaths.
> Fat resources can provide several days' worth of energy. Someone weighing 175 pounds with 15 percent body fat (about 26 pounds of body fat) is storing about 110,000 calories. In comparison, during a 90-minute workout, you might burn about 1,000 calories. So the fat you have is a virtually inexhaustible resource.
> Fat is about 60 percent of the brain's dry weight. Most brain fat is polyunsaturated fatty acids—structures containing two or more bonds, making the molecules pliable. They help maintain the flexibility of neurons, which transmit and receive information and maintain other functions of brain cells.

Contrary to popular belief, fats don't directly affect the accumulation of excess body fat or cause obesity. Instead, it is the imbalance of energy expenditure versus food consumption (whether in the form of excess fat, protein, or carbohydrates) that causes the deposition of energy reserves in subcutaneous adipose tissue. (The growth of fat cells is explained in Chapter 1.) A balanced and reasonable diet, tailored to the needs of the individual, minimizes the risk of accumulating excess body fat.

Different Fats Have Different Functions

Two basic types of lipids are found in cells: structural fats that form cell membranes and other structures, and neutral fats, which accumulate in fat cells

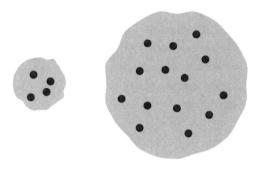

Fat cells grow in size, not in number.

and are converted to energy throughout the day. Structural fats are not used for energy production.

Fat in fat cells (adipocytes) undergoes continuous deconstruction and rebuilding (lipolysis and resynthesis, respectively). It is here that glucose is metabolized to fatty acids and, after the incorporation of glycerol, neutral fats are formed. These are broken down by lipase, and then the glycerol and free fatty acids formed in this reaction are released into the bloodstream.

A third type of fat is in brown fat cells. This tissue occurs in large quantities only in newborns and children, and it disappears with age. Its scant amounts in adults can be found on the back of the neck, in the abdomen, between the shoulder blades, and along the large vessels in the chest. Brown fat cells contain a lot of mitochondria, so they help to maintain the body's temperature.

CASE STUDY Fats Are Helpful and Necessary, Even for a Healthy Athlete

Meredith was a successful cyclist on a junior national team. She had improved over several years, but her performances eventually became stagnant. Tests on her body composition revealed that she wasn't properly balancing her nutrition with the demands of her sport. Without a nutritionist's consultation, Meredith had transitioned to an unbalanced diet with insufficient amounts of calories and fats. Consequently, she had reduced her level of body fat to 11 percent. Her poor diet also caused a decline in muscle mass, which translated into poor results in races and in training. Meredith stopped menstruating, but she considered it a normal side effect of competing at an elite level.

THE FIX: It was important for Meredith to learn about the role of fatty tissue in the body. Education was the first and most important step because without this awareness, she would not be inclined to increase the number of calories in her diet from both carbohydrates and healthy fats. Once she had this information, her fat intake was increased to 1 gram per kilogram of body weight per day, and her carbohydrate consumption was raised, too.

RESULTS: Meredith found that she began to feel better, and her performances improved, too. The changes to her diet helped improve her skin's appearance and restored her regular menstrual cycle. She was encouraged to maintain her healthy eating habits and to listen to her body, which translated into greater success on the bike. ■

Fat Classifications

Fats can also be categorized according to the number of double bonds in the fat molecule. All fatty acids found in food are divided into three groups:

> Saturated (no double bonds): Examples include palmitic acid and stearic acid.
> Monounsaturated (one double bond between a pair of carbon atoms): Examples include oleic acid and palmitoleic acid.
> Polyunsaturated (double bonds between more than one pair of carbon atoms): Examples include omega-6 and omega-3 fatty acids.

Yet another categorization of fats depends on the length of their carbon chains. There are short-, medium-, and long-chain fatty acids. Short-chain fatty acids contain fewer than 6 carbon atoms, medium-chain fatty acids have 6–10, and long-chain fatty acids have more than 12. Short- and medium-chain fatty acids in foods are less abundant than long-chain, but they are important for faster and easier digestion of the long-chain fats. Short-chain fatty acids are found in milk or butter fats, among other foods, whereas long-chain fatty acids appear in all fats of plant and animal origin.

Essential Fatty Acids

Essential fatty acids (EFAs) belong to the polyunsaturated group. The term "essential" is used to emphasize the need for these acids in our diet: Our body doesn't have enzymes that can create them, so we need to acquire them from what we eat. If we provide the essential fatty acids through food, other fatty acids can be formed from them. In particular, the omega-3 fatty acids found in fish are known to have many benefits:

> Substantial reduction in the concentration of triglycerides in blood plasma
> Regulation of blood pressure
> Reduction in blood platelets' susceptibility to clotting (acting as an anticoagulant)
> Strengthening of the immune system
> Prevention of hardening and narrowing of the arteries
> Anti-inflammatory and antiallergic properties and inhibition of the development of type 2 diabetes
> Antidepressant effects, supporting the proper functioning of the nerve cell membranes in the brain cortex
> Inhibition of lipogenesis, which is the formation of triglycerides using fatty acids, and thus counteracting obesity
> Support of the skin's hydration and reduction of acne

It's important to maintain a desirable ratio of omega-6 to omega-3 fatty acids, which should be below 4 to 1. In our modern Western society, this ratio has skyrocketed to as high as 20 to 1, bringing with it the effects of chronic diseases that follow such an intake.

Trans Fats

Trans fats are not found in plants or animals but rather created by a chemical process that converts naturally occurring liquid fats to a more solid form. They are ubiquitous in prepared foods. In products that include some sort of shortening (as is needed in baked goods), they appear nearly 90 percent of the time. These fats are also pervasive in ready-made meals and fast food. Because trans fats are slow to oxidize, they can be used for foods that need a long shelf life or when a fat must stand up to repeated exposure to the high temperatures of frying. Whether sourced from vegetable or animal fats, trans fats are one of the causes of health problems.

LOW LEVELS OF ESSENTIAL FATTY ACIDS CAN CAUSE MANY PROBLEMS

A lack of EFAs can disrupt many physiological functions. In the case of energy and nutrition, it can lead to the following problems:

> Limitations of ATP construction in mitochondria
> Cholesterol transport disorders
> Disorders in lipoproteins of cell membranes
> Increased cholesterol in the body
> Increased susceptibility to bacterial infections
> Disorders of many tissues and organs
> Deterioration of visual acuity
> Low muscle tone
> Excessive appetite
> Poor nitrogen retention in the body
> Reduced resistance to X-rays

Other negative effects include lack of weight gain, pathological kidney growth, enlargement of the heart muscle, and various skin changes.

Saturated Fats

Naturally occurring animal fats, found primarily in animal meats, raise the risk of high cholesterol, a condition that can cause many serious cardiovascular problems. But while animal fats increase total cholesterol in the blood, they balance the "bad" (LDL) and "good" (HDL) cholesterol levels, so the ratio of the two types doesn't fluctuate; only the overall quantity of the cholesterols changes.

The amount of saturated fatty acids (for example, bacon fat) should be limited in the diet because they increase the concentration of LDL cholesterol and triglycerides in the blood, which is known as one of the causes of cardio-vascular disease. As clinical studies have shown, one way to reduce saturated fat (from dairy products and meat) in the diet is to replace these fats with polyunsaturated fats from vegetable oils, which will reduce the risk of cardio-vascular disease.

When you remove saturated fats from your diet, it matters what you replace them with. Some studies have shown that, as a result of replacing saturated fats with refined carbohydrates (such as processed foods and soda), health complications can be significant and bring on an elevated risk of circulatory diseases. It's not enough to limit the saturated fatty acids in your diet; replace them with healthy foods, as well as adequate amounts of antioxidants.

Saturated fats are also found in a healthy configuration, an example of which is conjugated linoleic acid (CLA). It has very strong antioxidant properties that reduce both the formation of free radicals and the undesirable oxidation of lipids. Numerous studies have reported that some CLAs can play a part in weight loss because they inhibit the buildup of fat and also encourage the use of fat as an energy source; as we explained in Chapter 1, fats serve as a primary energy source in aerobic exercise. The best source of CLAs in the daily diet is milk, and more specifically, milk fat; substantially fewer CLAs appear in meats. Other benefits of CLAs include the following:

> Reduced susceptibility to atherosclerosis
> Accelerated reduction of body fat
> Antioxidant effects
> Inhibition of the development of type 2 diabetes
> Improved bone mineralization

Milk fat contains more than a dozen bioactive components with antioxidant properties, which play an important role in ensuring the balance between prooxidative and antioxidant activity. One study of 1,200 children aged 1–16 years showed that the children who were drinking skim milk were five times more likely to have gastroenteritis than those who drank whole milk. Milk fat supports the functions of the intestinal epithelium thanks to the short- and medium-chain saturated fatty acids that are derived from the fat in milk and produced by bacteria in the gut. These fats protect against bacterial toxins and rotaviruses, pathogens that cause gastroenteritis.

Medium-Chain Fats Preserve Some of Your Glycogen

Other healthy saturated fats recommended for the athlete are medium-chain triglycerides (MCTs). They are used to save carbohydrate reserves as a full-fledged source of energy for working muscles, and they can also increase the endurance of the muscles, delay their fatigue, and increase their strength. MCTs can also contribute to weight loss because they do not accumulate in adipose tissue, but they do accelerate the rate of metabolism.

MCTs in their natural form are found in coconut oil and coconut milk. Nutritional supplements offer these MCTs in more concentrated forms.

Fats During Exercise

How the body uses fat for energy production is affected by the intensity and duration of exercise, as well as the ease of the fat's mobility and oxidation. Fats are used primarily in medium- or low-intensity efforts, as discussed in Chapter 1. One kilogram (2.2 pounds) of adipose tissue could provide the energy needs for about 20 hours of running at an intensity of 60–70 percent VO_2max (maximum oxygen consumption). During endurance training with low intensity

SOME FACTS ABOUT COCONUT OIL

Coconut oil is credited with many health benefits, including improved athletic performance and post-workout recovery. Coconut's popularity extends beyond the food aisle; advocates claim it can act as sun protection and relieve bug bites. With such a plethora of coconut products and health claims, it's important to understand the science behind coconut oil.

First, coconut oil is a fat, so it plays less of a role in recovery compared to carbohydrates and protein. Second, it belongs to a group of saturated fats that our body needs, but in a smaller proportion to the other fatty acids.

Third, about 60 percent of coconut oil is lauric acid, which is quite beneficial and is present in similar proportions only in breast milk. The body transforms lauric acid into compounds with antibacterial and antiviral properties. This acid, unlike antibiotics, does not affect the naturally occurring bacterial flora that is crucial to our health.

Fourth, coconut oil contains medium-chain triglycerides (MCT), which are digested and metabolized in a completely different way from other fats. Instead of storing them in fat cells, the body uses them to produce energy, which stimulates and accelerates the body's overall metabolism. However, the content of MCT in coconut products is only about 10 percent, so it does not significantly affect the rate of metabolism.

Finally, coconut oil has a high smoking point, making it ideal for cooking foods at high temperatures without compromising your health and without changing the flavor of the meal.

Coconut oil has its benefits, but it is no cure-all. It can be included in your daily meal plan, but remember that it is a fat—and in fact, a saturated fat—so we should consume it in limited quantities to maintain the balance of lipids in our body.

(50 percent VO$_2$max), about 75 percent of the energy comes from fat, while the remainder comes from carbohydrates and a negligible amount from protein.

Fat is also burned during other efforts, including strength training: The start of physical exercise causes the expansion of small blood vessels, which significantly contributes to the easier supply of free fatty acids to working muscles, where they are used as energy. Therefore, in almost every type of exercise (except for efforts using the phosphagen system mentioned in Chapter 1), the body uses fat, but sometimes its quantities are minimal—even just a few grams.

 How long should I exercise to start burning fat?

Oxygen-based energy production, including the use of fat, starts after a few minutes of effort. In the beginning of an aerobic workout, fat contributions are indeed small. Greater use of fats will come with longer workouts, as explained in Chapter 1, so to be sure you've asked your body to burn a fair amount of fat, it is worth running at least 30 minutes, or preferably longer.

Optimal Body Fat Content

Knowing that fats are important, but that too much of the wrong fats can be problematic and unnecessary, you might ask how much body fat you should have. When it comes to the question of an ideal body fat composition, it's hard to identify a simple rule because it depends on many factors, including sex, age, and level of activity. Athletes present a particular challenge because their optimal body composition also depends on their sport; large muscle mass or very little body fat reserves are not always recommended. The performance level in the athlete's sport is also significant: Ideal composition will look different for the amateur compared to the professional. Some general guidelines can apply, though.

In high-performance female athletes aged 17–25, the optimal fat content can be about 12–16 percent (or depending on body shape, up to 20 percent).

In female athletes aged 25–35, it can be 4–5 percent higher. Women who do not participate in sports should be in the range of 20–25 percent. In male professional athletes aged 15–25, the optimal fat levels can be 7–13 percent, and in ages 25–35, up to 16 percent. Men in their 20s and 30s who don't exercise should aim for less than 20 percent body fat.

In some sports, athletes lower their fat composition to the lowest possible level. Professional bodybuilders might try to drop their fat content to 5 percent during certain periods, while professional female cyclists, dancers, gymnasts, and general fitness athletes sometimes have less than 10 percent body fat. These levels can present a high risk of health problems because fat tissue truly is necessary for us, and it is particularly important for women. Many female athletes with poor energy levels and suboptimal body fat percentage can develop hormone-management problems, which often manifests in the absence of menstruation. As a result, this condition can ultimately lead to infertility as well as other complications like osteoporosis, injury, and illness.

Can I use a body mass index calculator to see how fit I am?

The body mass index (BMI) estimates whether a person is below, at, or above ideal weight. It's a measure of your weight according to height, but it is limited in its accuracy because it does not discern between fat and muscle and other components of the body. Nor does it consider your level of physical activity, and if you do exercise, to what extent or intensity.

The BMI standard ranges from 18.5 to 24.9. Below 18.5 is considered underweight, and above 25 is overweight (over 30 signifies obesity). But consider bodybuilders, who maintain a low body fat composition and have a large amount of muscle mass, contributing to more body weight. According to the BMI ranges, they would turn out to be quite overweight. So BMI estimates can be misleading. The entire composition of the body (body fat, water, muscle, and so on) is always important, not only the body weight and height.

TABLE 4.1 Cholesterol content in selected foods

Food		Cholesterol Content (milligrams per 100 grams of food)
Egg yolk	>	1,085
Fish oil	>	490
Liver	>	350
Butter	>	215
Cheese	>	100
Cream (30% fat)	>	100
Cow milk (2% fat)	>	8
Yogurt/kefir	>	6–8

Cholesterol

Cholesterol is found in all body cells, and it is particularly important for the nervous and endocrine systems. The human body is able to create cholesterol in most cells, but a large supply of energy is needed to create cholesterol, so about 30 percent of it comes from the food we eat.

Both diet and the efficiency of individual hormones affect the amount of cholesterol we store. In most cases, cholesterol supplied from food has little effect on its concentration in the blood. Cholesterol is found in animal products in various concentrations (see Table 4.1).

"Good" and "Bad" Cholesterol

We often speak of cholesterol in terms of HDL and LDL, and technically, these are not types of cholesterol but the carriers responsible for its transport in our body. LDL is low-density lipoprotein, commonly referred to as "bad" cholesterol. When there's too much of it, large amounts of cholesterol accumulate in the cells of the arterial walls, creating deposits called atherosclerotic

TABLE 4.2 LDL cholesterol ranges for men and women

LDL Level (milligrams per deciliter of blood)		Assessment
Below 100	>	Optimal
100–129	>	Above optimal
130–159	>	Borderline high
160–189	>	High
>190	>	Very high

TABLE 4.3 HDL cholesterol ranges for men and women

HDL Level (milligrams per deciliter of blood)		Assessment
35 (men) 40 (women)	>	HDL levels below these thresholds pose a high risk of heart disease
60	>	At or above this level is considered healthy

plaques. These can calcify and harden over time. As the deposits develop, the blood vessel's interior narrows and limits the body's ability to move blood—containing nutrients and oxygen—throughout the body. Organs then lose some of their efficiency.

Cholesterols formed in the body and those acquired through food are involved in the formation of atherosclerotic plaques. An improper diet with a high proportion of unhealthy fats, carbohydrates, and cholesterol increases LDL levels. Trans fatty acids, too, can increase LDL cholesterol while lowering HDL cholesterol levels, an imbalance that can cause many diseases and complications. A blood test can reveal the amount of LDL in your body, measured in milligrams per deciliter of blood (one tenth of a liter), and whether it is at a desirable level (see Table 4.2).

TABLE 4.4 Interpreting a blood test's total cholesterol level

Total Cholesterol Level (milligrams per deciliter of blood)		Assessment
<200	>	Desired, healthy value
200–239	>	Borderline high
>240	>	High; presents increased risk of heart disease

HDL is high-density lipoprotein, known as the "good" cholesterol. It can remove cholesterol from the walls of blood vessels. A high level of HDL is considered to be beneficial to our health (see Table 4.3). The lower limit of the norm is 35 milligrams per deciliter of blood, while the upper limit is not specified. For women, this level should be slightly higher. Research has shown that values above 70 milligrams per deciliter are particularly helpful in reducing the risk of cardiovascular diseases.

Despite the generally accepted opinion that serum cholesterol increases with age, research has shown that it depends mainly on nutrition, lifestyle, physical activity, and genetic conditions. Cholesterol is important for the endocrine and nervous systems, and it also takes part in the formation of bile acids (for digestion) and vitamins A, D3, E, and K.

Studies have shown that on average a man consumes approximately 34 percent of calories from fat. On a 2,000–3,000 calorie diet, that's an intake of about 75–115 grams of fat and 340 milligrams of cholesterol each day. Up to 25–30 percent of a food's cholesterol can be absorbed via the intestine, but the amount depends mainly on the activity of the secreted bile and to a lesser extent the content of cholesterol and fat in the food. Research suggests that reducing the cholesterol doses in food only slightly affects its serum concentration and improvement in lipid levels in the blood. And interestingly, it's believed that the development of atherosclerosis depends more on long-term deficiencies of antioxidants than the amount of fat in the diet. Blood tests can reveal your cholesterol count; the value will fall into one of a few levels of risk (see Table 4.4).

High-Fat Diets

In the 1990s, a few high-fat diets became very popular. They promoted the consumption of foods containing high levels of fat and the exclusion or extreme limitation of carbohydrates. It was thought that pork, lard, butter, fatty sauces, and cheese could be eaten to no end. The recommended proportions were in the range of 1.0 grams of protein to 2.5–3.5 grams of fat to 0.5 grams of carbohydrate. Such a balance was supposed to improve health and well-being and paradoxically reduce body fat (up to 10 pounds per month). It is true that a

---

DO EGGS CAUSE THE ONSET OF CARDIOVASCULAR DISEASE OR DIABETES?

For years, the consumption of cholesterol-containing eggs had been at the center of controversy. A theory took root claiming that an excess of eggs (specifically their yolks) promotes the deposition of "bad" cholesterol, and thus poses a threat to the cardiovascular system. In one of many studies to examine this relationship, 22 independent groups were examined, divided into people consuming at least one egg per day and those eating up to one egg per week. From the results of the study, it was concluded that egg consumption is not associated with the risk of cardiovascular disease and mortality in the general population.

As the prevalence of type 2 diabetes increases worldwide, studies have also been conducted to show whether eggs are associated with the incidence of this disease. It is known that eggs are a substantial source of cholesterol, which is associated with an increased level of glucose in the blood, and this in turn increases the risk of type 2 diabetes. One investigation of this relationship involved 2,332 men aged 42–60. It turned out that the consumption of chicken eggs is associated with a very low risk of type 2 diabetes. Subsequent studies have further demonstrated that the consumption of eggs is not connected to the disease.

high-fat diet (with a drastic reduction in carbohydrates) contributes to the reduction of body fat. However, numerous scientific studies have confirmed that if someone follows this diet for a long time (often for many years), he or she significantly increases the risk of atherosclerosis and mortality from cardiovascular diseases. Excessive fat consumption, often containing "bad" cholesterol, and the lack of physical activity can lead to extreme, even dangerous accumulation of fats around internal organs. And not only the kidneys, liver, and stomach, but also the heart and blood vessels, which bring on other health problems.

This diet, though it still has its supporters, is criticized today because, in light of current research, the main source of calories should be grains, vegetables, fruits, milk and milk products, lean meat, and fish—not predominately animal fats.

Ketogenic Diets

The principles of the high-fat diet now appear in a new form: the ketogenic diet. These diet plans rely on fats as the primary source of energy and nutrition. Ketogenic diets promote the consumption of vegetable fats (oils,

---

THE BIG PICTURE OF HUMAN HEALTH

About 60 nutrients are necessary for humans, including 10 essential amino acids, 1–4 essential unsaturated fatty acids, 1–2 sugars, 21 minerals, and 18 vitamins. The diet should also contain fiber from vegetables. All of these elements should be delivered daily in multiple meals because metabolic processes require a constant supply of energy and individual nutrients. Without them, some biochemical, functional, or even morphological changes may occur, possibly manifesting themselves in abnormal physical and mental development and changes to tissues, organs, or entire systems of the body.

pumpkin seeds, sunflower seeds, and avocados, for example), fish and animal fats, and some protein. Some of these diets limit carbohydrates to levels as low as 25–50 grams per day.

The ketogenic diet was originally used to help people with epilepsy. This high-fat and moderate-protein diet with carbohydrates well below 50 grams per day encourages the body to source energy from fats by way of ketone bodies rather than carbohydrates. Ketone bodies are constantly produced by the body, usually at the average of 0.1 millimole per deciliter. With the absence of carbohydrates in a ketogenic diet, the body is prompted to use more ketones and fat for energy—at least 0.5 millimole of ketone bodies per deciliter, and according to other sources, 0.2 millimole per deciliter.

The proportions between macronutrients are important to encourage ketosis: 70–75 percent of calories should come from fat, about 20 percent from protein, and 5–10 percent from carbohydrates, mainly in the form of fibrous foods, in order to arrive at a reduced level of "net carbohydrates." With such a low intake of carbohydrates, the level of glucose and insulin in the blood drops significantly, and the body begins to use the stored fat, which gets into the liver, where it is then metabolized in the process of beta-oxidation (decomposition of fatty acids). Further discussion of the ketogenic diet and a sample meal plan are presented in Chapter 6, "Sample Meal Plans."

Nutrition Roundup

Fats are indispensable in the athlete's diet. They are involved in many important processes: the construction of cell membranes, the absorption of some vitamins, hormonal balance, energy production at low and moderate intensity, and body temperature control.

Fats provide energy primarily in low-intensity physical efforts, such as a run of a few miles or more, or a long bike ride. The longer your effort, the more fat you burn. Heavy perspiration (sweat) during exercise has little to do with fat reduction.

Cholesterol is a naturally occurring substance in our body, categorized into "bad" (LDL) and "good" (HDL) types. When the LDL level is too high, it is deposited in the cells of the arterial walls, creating deposits called atherosclerotic plaques, which lead to dangerous narrowing of the arteries. The task of HDL is to remove cholesterol from the walls of blood vessels. A high level of HDL is considered beneficial to health.

Recommended Fat Intake

Guidelines for daily fat consumption are often calculated according to a person's total daily caloric intake.

	Daily Fat Intake			
Typical Daily Caloric Intake	Fat as 20% of Total Calories		Fat as 35% of Total Calories	
	(calories)	(grams)	(calories)	(grams)
1,500 >	300	33	525	58
1,600 >	320	35	560	62
1,700 >	340	37	595	65
1,800 >	360	40	630	69
1,900 >	380	42	665	73
2,000 >	400	44	700	77
2,100 >	420	46	735	81
2,200 >	440	48	770	85
2,300 >	460	51	805	88
2,400 >	480	53	840	92
2,500 >	500	55	875	96
2,600 >	520	57	910	100
2,700 >	540	59	945	104
2,800 >	560	62	980	108

Continues

Continued

Daily Fat Intake

Typical Daily Caloric Intake		Fat as 20% of Total Calories		Fat as 35% of Total Calories	
		(calories)	(grams)	(calories)	(grams)
2,900	>	580	64	1,015	112
3,000	>	600	66	1,050	115
3,100	>	620	68	1,085	119
3,200	>	640	70	1,120	123
3,300	>	660	73	1,155	127
3,400	>	680	75	1,190	131
3,500	>	700	77	1,225	135
3,600	>	720	79	1,260	138
3,700	>	740	81	1,295	142

Note: Recommended fat consumption is calculated as a percentage of total caloric intake, ranging from 20% to 35% of total calories.

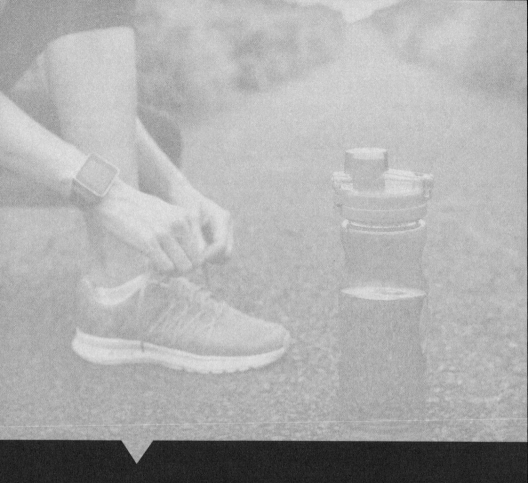

5 HYDRATION

Water can constitute up to 55 percent of body weight in women and up to 60 percent of body weight in men (and slightly more in athletes). About 55 percent of the total water contained in the body is found inside cells, about 39 percent in intercellular fluids, and the remaining 6 percent in plasma and lymph.

The demand for water of a healthy adult is about 40 grams per kilogram of body weight, or about 4 percent of body weight per day. Interestingly, in infants, the daily water demand is much higher, at about 100 grams per kilogram of body weight or 10 percent of body weight.

We lose water not only during exercise and physical work, but also during rest. Water losses also occur as a result of physiological processes throughout the day. Excluding losses during physical exercise, a person loses 2,200–2,600 milliliters of water each day through urine (1,300–1,500 mL), the skin (500–600 mL), the lungs (300–400 mL), and feces (approximately 100 mL). The average person consumes water in the form of liquids (1,300–1,500 mL); with food, mainly vegetables (700–800 mL); and through metabolic changes (200–300 mL); all of which more or less makes up for all the water that's lost.

In the case of athletes, the loss of liquids will be significantly higher. This is due to, in part, the increase of the metabolic rate during exercise—up to 20 times greater than resting metabolism. Therefore, the rate of heat generation increases, and in the first few minutes, the temperature in working muscles reaches up to 102°F (at rest, muscle temperatures are near 93°F–96°F). The entire body will rise in temperature, and the heat is dispersed through several mechanisms of thermoregulation: conduction, radiation, convection, and evaporation of sweat from the skin surface.

The first three methods make up the so-called dry heat exchange, which can account for about 70 percent of all heat loss in a cool and dry environment. However, if the air temperature is higher than 95°F, the excess heat can be released only by the fourth method: evaporation. Increased physical activity results in sweat production of up to 1.5 liters during one training session, but if the effort is performed on a hot and steamy day, sweat loss can be up to 4 liters per hour. Just sitting in a warm room or outdoor area accelerates breathing such that the water loss through exhaled air can reach as much as

1,500–2,000 milliliters. Some athletes hardly sweat at all, while others produce up to 4–5 liters of sweat during intense training. Perspiration depends mainly on the weight and composition of the body, but also on sex, age, and fitness level.

Sweat removes not only water but also electrolytes such as sodium, chlorine, potassium, and magnesium and in smaller amounts, calcium, iron, copper, bicarbonates, phosphates, sulfates, amino acids, and some vitamins. Of course, the rate of excretion of sweat is individually variable.

Sometimes athletes and coaches think heavy sweating is undesirable, but in fact, in a well-trained athlete, it's a sign not of weakness but of an efficiently functioning thermoregulatory system. If physical exercise is performed in a hot or humid environment, heat dissipation is very difficult. The expulsion of 1 liter of sweat causes the loss of 2.9 grams of sodium chloride, so athletes training intensely lose about 15 grams of salt with every 5 liters of sweat. (Some recommendations for daily salt intake among the general population are therefore lower than what's best for an athlete.)

Some athletes have problems getting rid of excess heat. Their bodies overheat, their faces become red, and they might have to stop or slow down their pace. This is caused by a disorder of sweat production, which may be due to many factors such as obesity, sleep deficiency, an overactive thyroid, and also some medicines, including fever-reducers, psychotropics, sedatives, antihistamines, and beta-blockers used to treat hypertension.

 What can I do to manage body heat on a really hot day?

Especially on hot and humid days of competition, some athletes prepare their bodies for efficient heat regulation by pre-cooling. It involves lowering the skin and internal temperature to prevent overheating during exercise. The most popular methods are bathing in cold water, taking a cold shower, and wearing ice jackets or vests. It's advised to use these methods only with guidance from a professional trainer.

Maintaining Hydration

Even just a few generations ago, up to the 1970s, athletes were advised not to drink any fluids during exercise due to the potential load on the digestive system and a negative impact on exercise capacity. Years later, the advice flip-flopped: Athletes were told to take on a lot of fluids to counteract dehydration and overheating. With the recommendation going from one extreme to the other, the problem became not dehydration but overhydration. Extreme hydration can cause serious complications, including hyponatremia (a deficiency of sodium in the blood), which can lead to death. There is a healthy middle ground.

The correct amount of fluids in the diet depends on many factors:

Age: Adults require more fluids than teens and children.

Sex: On average, men require more fluids than women because of greater muscle mass.

Temperature and humidity: More fluids are needed when it's hot and humid.

Type of physical activity: Exertion can raise fluid requirements toward 10 liters per day.

Health problems: Increased hydration is advised for fevers, diabetes, thyroid disorders, and illness involving diarrhea or vomiting.

Type of diet: High-protein, high-sodium, and high-carbohydrate diets require greater hydration.

Some athletes assess their hydration levels based on the volume and color of their urine. Dark yellow urine means that the body is very dehydrated and requires immediate replenishment of fluids. A bright yellow color indicates a high degree of dehydration; yellow, a moderate degree of dehydration; light yellow, acceptable hydration; and clear, colorless urine means that the level of fluids in the body is good.

A more accurate method of determining hydration levels—although not applicable for everyday use—is the measurement of urine density using an

THE IMPORTANCE OF KIDNEYS IN FLUIDS REGULATION

The kidneys are responsible for maintaining the balance of water in body fluids, which supports normal cell membrane structure and cell function. Excess water and inorganic compounds such as sodium, potassium, chlorine, and calcium are removed from the blood via the kidneys. The body is well prepared to regulate water and electrolytes, so even a significant rise in water and mineral salts from food does not disturb the balance of fluids. Efficient kidneys are the key to success in managing this balance, so healthy kidneys are important for athletes.

osmometer, which is best done in a laboratory. Osmolality is a picture of the concentration of sodium, potassium, chloride, glucose, and urea in plasma as well as in urine and feces. The higher the osmolality, the worse the hydration.

The sensation of thirst prompts the body to supplement about half the volume of lost fluids. However, thirst appears only after you've lost 1–2 percent of your fluids, which seems small but can significantly reduce athletic performance. Using thirst as an indicator of fluid demand can be misleading. And just as the feeling of thirst doesn't reflect the exact moment of fluid loss (it's too late, in fact), drinking enough to quench your thirst doesn't mean you've fully hydrated your body.

During exercise, fluids are lost through sweat but also through the normal functions of metabolism and in the kidneys and lungs. Each gram of glycogen binds about 2.7 grams of water, which is released during glycogen oxidation. During intense training, if we burn 1,200 calories with about 80 percent of the energy coming from muscle glycogen, 800 milliliters of water will be released. About 900 of the 1,200 calories will be removed from the body in the form of heat, if the body temperature is to remain unchanged. The elimination of 900 calories is associated with the evaporation of about 1.5 liters of water. This process, therefore, significantly contributes to the dehydration of the body.

Q How much water do I need each day?

The simplest way to calculate water demand is to assume that 1 milliliter of water is needed for every 1 calorie in your diet. For someone with a 2,000-calorie diet, 2 liters of water should be enough. A different method to determine water intake is to drink 300 milliliters for every 10 kilograms of body weight (22 lb). So, someone weighing 80 kilograms (175 lb) should drink about 2,400 milliliters, or 2.4 liters per day. These recommendations exclude the hydration requirements to recover from exercise, which are described in the questions below.

REFER TO THE WATER intake guidelines in Table 5.3 and on pp. 116–117 to see how much water is recommended according to your body weight.

Fluids come from not only water but also other food and drink, such as tea, coffee, fruit and vegetable juices (which are 85–95 percent water), milk and milk drinks (80–90 percent), soups and purees (70–96 percent), and fruits and vegetables (about 90 percent).

Q What can I do to be sure I'm hydrated before a workout?

Research has shown that the body needs 8–12 hours to replenish its hydration after an intense workout, assuming a balanced diet and proper hydration methods are followed. If there is less time between workouts or you haven't eaten or hydrated well, you can use an aggressive hydration plan: Drink about 2.25–3.1 milliliters of fluid per pound of body weight (for a person weighing 165 pounds, that equates to 375–511 milliliters) four hours before your workout. If you don't feel a need to urinate or the urine is dark and thick, take another 1.4–2.25 milliliters per pound of body weight two hours before training. The process can be supplemented with the addition of sodium: Take 360–900 milligrams per deciliter of water you drink or eat some small salty snacks. Either technique will increase thirst and facilitate the absorption of fluids.

A MINOR DROP IN FLUID LEVELS CAUSES MAJOR PROBLEMS

A loss of fluids causing a 2 percent drop in body weight (3.5 pounds for a 170-pound athlete) causes a 10 percent decrease in efficiency. That's substantial! In track and field sprinting, where hundredths of a second count, such a change can make a big difference in performance. Research published in 2017 by *Sports Medicine* shows that athletes in soccer, basketball, cricket, and baseball often lose up to 3–4 percent of body weight in fluids. The loss of 5 percent of the body's water causes many problems within the circulatory, respiratory, and muscular systems. Losing 15 percent of the body's water is usually fatal.

The balance of nutrients, electrolytes, and water is very important during post-workout recovery. Researchers found that up to 25 percent of triathletes and ultramarathoners taking part in competitions in the Caribbean suffer from hyponatremia—a sharp decline in sodium levels. It usually occurs four to six hours after the end of exercise and usually manifests itself as muscle cramps, confusion, mental block, and even epileptic seizures. There have also been reports of complete respiratory arrest as a result. Poor sodium levels are brought on primarily by the consumption of fluids that lack adequate sodium content during exercise. More details on healthy rehydration are discussed under "Sports Drinks and the Water-Nutrient Balance" (p. 102) and the hydration plan in Table 5.3 (p. 114).

To accurately monitor your water intake, you can track how much fluid you tend to lose during exercise and then replace that amount during and after the workout. And in fact, you should consume even more than the amount lost: between 150 and 200 percent of the fluids lost. To determine what you've lost, weigh yourself before and after training. If, after exercise, you weigh 1 kilogram (2.2 lb) less, you should drink about 1,500–2,000 milliliters of water in small doses (don't guzzle down 2 liters of water).

Not All Water Is the Same

Very little water that you drink contains solely H_2O. Most water, whether it comes from the tap, mountain springs, or any other source, contains other compounds. It's helpful to know what is—and is not—in your water because a healthy water supply does affect your body and your nutrition plan: What you don't get through water, you'll need to supply through other foods.

Mineral Water

Mineral water, to obtain such a label, should contain an appropriate amount of minerals and should be drawn from wells protected from external factors; it can't be treated or contain any additives.

The composition of mineral waters can vary. Most of the options available in stores contain 200–500 milligrams of micronutrients per liter of water. The US Food and Drug Administration mandates that products labeled "mineral water" must contain at least 250 parts per million of dissolved solids. Low mineral content is considered between 250 and 500 parts per million; bottles labeled "high mineral content" have more than 1,500 parts per million.

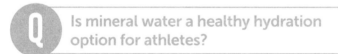

Q Is mineral water a healthy hydration option for athletes?

Active people can benefit from drinking highly mineralized water before, during, and after workouts because the losses of micro- and macronutrients during training can be substantial. The greatest attention should be paid to the content of potassium, magnesium, and bicarbonates because they help maintain the acid-base balance of the blood and avoid painful muscle cramps after training. However, this type of water should not be used all the time or in large quantities as it may lead to an excess of minerals. So drink waters with varying micronutrient content during the day.

If you have trouble digesting or your stomach becomes a little too acidic, then it might be helpful to drink water rich in bicarbonates (more than 500 milligrams per liter). Bicarbonates neutralize stomach acids, so they relieve stomachaches after meals. Magnesium will benefit athletes experiencing effects of overtraining or consuming large amounts of coffee; look for water with more than 50 milligrams per liter.

It is also worth paying attention to the sodium content (more than 200 milligrams per liter is recommended), especially if you are prone to excessive sweating; the losses of this mineral with sweat can be enormous. Sodium directly affects the body's water management, preventing dehydration. But for those with elevated blood pressure, low-sodium water is more appropriate.

In weight-loss diets, it is usually advised to drink a lot of liquids. So choose water with a high content of calcium and magnesium to cleanse the body of toxins, as the increased levels of these minerals enhance the filtration mechanisms of the kidneys.

Spring Water

Natural spring water contains small amounts of minerals (less than 500 milligrams per liter). It is suitable for everyday consumption, including for children and the elderly. Many people drink spring water either directly or after filtering it; however, it should be remembered that drinking such water for a long time may cause disturbance of water and electrolyte management. This depends on the water source and intake, composition, and quality.

Distilled Water

Sometimes athletes will experiment with less common approaches to nutrition or hydration. Among those experiments has been the use of distilled water, especially in strength or bodybuilding sports. This is the same water that is used for ironing clothing and in car radiators, in fact. Distilled water does not provide the body with any nutrients, unlike mineral water or even tap water, so it can, as a result of osmosis, draw out helpful compounds like electrolytes from the body. Such a loss of nutrients is eventually harmful.

Distilled water can actually dehydrate the body, and for this reason, some people drink it to prompt specific changes in their body. In bodybuilding, it's mainly used before a competition to get rid of even a few hundred milliliters of liquids within a short time so that the athlete can stay within a weight category or to dehydrate the body in order to make muscles more visible. But drinking distilled water can be very harmful to your health.

Q Does carbonated water affect me as an athlete?

Drinking carbonated, seltzer, or sparkling water isn't advised during exercise because it provides more carbon dioxide, which your body is trying to remove—and at a faster rate when you're breathing heavily. Carbonated water doesn't adequately quench thirst—it actually suppresses thirst—and causes bloating (especially in people with gastric problems). It disrupts the body's electrolyte balance, particularly in people with kidney disease. This kind of water reduces the lungs' ability to efficiently remove gasses from the body, and it worsens dehydration. Carbonated water isn't recommended for those suffering from hyperacidity, peptic ulcer disease, or problems in the throat or larynx. A time when carbonated water can be consumed is after exercise because it accelerates the excretion of harmful by-products from the body.

Sports Drinks and the Water-Nutrient Balance

Sports and energy drinks will contain different proportions of electrolytes compared to the blood's composition of the same compounds. How the concentrations in the drink and the blood compare will affect the body's hydration and nutrient balance. A drink that has a lower concentration of compounds than the concentration in the body is called *hypotonic*. A drink with higher concentrations is *hypertonic*. And when the beverage and blood have the same concentrations, the drink is *isotonic*. Each of these are appropriate for an athlete, but the quantity and time of consumption matters.

Depending on their ingredients, sports drinks could fall into any of these three categories. Some are labeled with their type, but many are not. Most of the more common drinks fall into the isotonic category, but check the nutrition label to know how many carbs are in a serving. Specific ranges of carbohydrate composition in each type of tonic are presented in the sections that follow.

Hypotonic Drinks

Hypotonic liquids encourage the fastest transfer of water into the body. These drinks include water and other diluted drinks that contain lower concentrations of minerals and other ingredients than the concentration in the body (for example, some vegetable and fruit juices). Equally important, these liquids contain only a small amount of carbohydrates (less than 4 grams per 100 milliliters).

Because these drinks are quickly absorbed through the gastrointestinal tract, if consumed in high quantities they can dilute the plasma and prompt more frequent urination, thereby decreasing overall hydration levels. Drinking plain water during a long, intense effort is not enough to properly hydrate the body, as some of the electrolytes can move into the gastrointestinal tract, causing hyponatremia. On hot days, sweat losses are high, and while the body needs more water, it's important to add in electrolytes, too.

Isotonic Drinks

Isotonics have a nearly identical composition as our body fluids. The carbohydrate content is in the range of 4–8 grams per 100 milliliters, and the minerals are close to the composition of sweat. Isotonic drinks provide electrolytes and glucose, which lets you save or supplement muscle glycogen. Therefore, these types of beverages are recommended during training lasting over 60 minutes or immediately afterward, to compensate for losses. They are especially important if your workout involves a lot of high-intensity effort, when glycogen and electrolytes are lost quickly. Remember that if you drink electrolyte-rich isotonics, you should not also reach for highly mineralized water; instead, take water with low levels of minerals, like spring water. In addition, isotonic drinks should not be consumed as a substitute for other drinks during the day, such as tea or juices, especially by kids and teens.

When the goal of your training is to reduce body fat, avoid these isotonic drinks during a workout so that you can encourage your body to draw energy from body fat.

Coconut Water

A "natural isotonic" is found inside the coconut. It has similar concentrations of sugar and electrolytes as our body fluids. And it contains large amounts of B vitamins, amino acids, and enzymes. Some doctors recommend it to people who have kidney stones because it is a natural diuretic, increasing the production of urine.

Coconut water contains a variety of minerals (see Table 5.1). The composition of ions contained in coconut water can help replenish electrolytes such as potassium, calcium, and magnesium, which are all lost through sweat during physical exercise or in hot climates. With such properties, coconut water can be used as a natural isotonic drink. In addition, it has been shown that the high potassium content contributes to proper heart function.

Hypertonic Drinks

Hypertonic liquids include fruit juices, highly sweetened beverages, and other carbohydrate-heavy drinks. The concentration of minerals and vitamins is higher than in body fluids, and the carbohydrate content exceeds 8 grams per 100 milliliters. They are helpful because they provide many nutrients that were lost during exercise, but they draw water from the body and into the intestines, and they reduce the rate of rehydration. This means that your cells, which need water, have in fact lost some hydration.

Hypertonic drinks taken during intense physical exercise may cause gastrointestinal distress, nausea, and diarrhea. These types of drinks cause a rapid increase in blood sugar levels, leading to hyperglycemia. The pancreas then responds quickly, releasing insulin and reducing blood-sugar levels, almost causing a hypoglycemic condition. Over the long term, such fluctuations in blood sugar can lead to insulin resistance.

TABLE 5.1 **Coconut water offers many minerals and vitamins**

		Quantity in 100 grams of Coconut Water
Energy	>	24 cal
Carbohydrates	>	4.8 g
Protein	>	0.72 g
Fat	>	0.2 g
Calcium	>	24–31.64 mg
Magnesium	>	6.4–30 mg
Potassium	>	203.7–312 mg
Sodium	>	1.75–105 mg
Thiamine (B1)	>	0.03 mg
Riboflavin (B2)	>	0.057 mg
Niacin (B3)	>	0.08 mg
Pantothenic acid (B5)	>	0.043 mg
Pyridoxine (B6)	>	0.032 mg
Folate	>	0.03 mg

Energy Drinks

Energy drinks are becoming more and more popular in sports and beyond; they've been around since the 1960s, in fact. Today's energy drinks can contain a long list of ingredients, including caffeine, guarana, taurine, inositol, carbohydrates, B vitamins, and ginseng root extract.

Energy drinks are designed for physically active people and contain ingredients that improve reaction time, concentration, and efficiency of the body. They improve metabolism and counteract the sensation of fatigue.

Be cautious when choosing these drinks. Many of their active ingredients can interfere with the body's biochemical processes, so they can sometimes be toxic (see Table 5.2). Energy drinks are particularly discouraged for children and adolescents, while it's estimated that in the United States, 31 percent of youth aged 12–17 consume them.

Research has consistently documented such drinks' adverse effects. In one study, nine energy drinks were examined to assess their acidification of the body (they lower pH levels), buffering capacity, and sugar content. These beverages were found to promote high acidity, which in combination with a high carbohydrate content (mainly sucrose) can damage tooth enamel. Other

TABLE 5.2 **Composition of popular energy drinks**

Drink Brand	Caffeine Content (mg per 100 ml of drink)	Calorie Content (calories per 100 ml of drink)	Other Ingredients
Monster Energy	33	46	Sugar; glucose; citric acid; taurine; panax ginseng extract; L-carnitine L-tartrate; vitamins B2, B3, B6, B12; inositol; guarana extract
NOS	34–55	42	High fructose corn syrup; taurine; caffeine; L-theanine; sucralose; vitamins B6, B12; guarana extract
Rockstar	33	58	Taurine, maltodextrin, guarana seed extract, L-carnitine, inositol, milk thistle extract, ginkgo biloba leaf extract, B vitamins, *Eleutherococcus senticosus*
Red Bull	32	45	Taurine, glucuronolactone, caffeine, B group vitamins, inositol
Red Bull Energy Shot	133	45	Taurine, glucuronolactone, caffeine, B group vitamins, inositol

studies have shown that the consumption of energy drinks 60 minutes before training indeed improves muscle strength, but it also causes insomnia and nervousness after the effort.

Other Caffeinated Beverages

Caffeine is a chemical (an alkaloid) that occurs naturally in the leaves, grains, and fruits of several dozen plant species around the world. It is found in products such as tea, coffee, and many other nonalcoholic beverages. Caffeine is known for its stimulating effect, which is often used to combat fatigue or sleepiness, but it also causes insomnia in people highly sensitive to it. Because caffeine enters the bloodstream relatively quickly, the psychostimulant effect

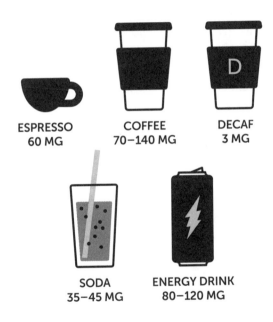

ESPRESSO
60 MG

COFFEE
70–140 MG

DECAF
3 MG

SODA
35–45 MG

ENERGY DRINK
80–120 MG

Caffeine content shown applies to 1 oz. espresso and 12 oz. coffee and soda. Many energy drinks come in 250-milliliter cans, so drinking the entire can would provide 80–120 milligrams of caffeine.

occurs equally quickly and can last several hours. Each person responds to caffeine differently, according to our metabolism, body mass, muscle mass, age, and sex. It's been long believed that caffeine will dehydrate the body, but recent research demonstrates that although it has a small diuretic effect, it doesn't cause dehydration.

Extreme consumption of caffeinated drinks can be dangerous, but the lethal dose of caffeine for an adult is quite high: 200–400 milligrams per kilogram of body weight, which on average means consumption of 10–12 grams of pure caffeine, or drinking 30 liters of an energy drink.

Caffeine is absorbed along almost the entire length of the digestive system, from the stomach, through the small and large intestines, and in the rectum; it is metabolized in the liver. Total absorption into the blood occurs after about 45 minutes, and the maximum concentration in the blood serum can remain up to two or three hours after drinking it, although it varies individually.

Caffeine also has an effect on the mood and behavior of children and adolescents. A team of Canadian scientists determined a daily recommended dose of caffeine for children aged 4–6 years should be no more than 45 milligrams; 7–9 years, a maximum of 62 milligrams; and 10–12 years, up to 85 milligrams. Research has shown that 73 percent of adolescents aged 12–18 consume at least 100 milligrams of caffeine per day, mainly in the afternoon, which may negatively affect their sleep.

Green Coffee

Green coffee has become increasingly popular—especially among people trying to lose extra weight. Studies have found that it supports health in several ways, such as aiding with weight loss, lowering blood pressure, and controlling blood sugar. Green coffee is simply coffee brewed with unroasted beans. It contains less caffeine than roasted beans (about 24 milligrams in an 8-ounce cup), and it provides a substantial amount of chlorogenic acid, which is the key source of green coffee's beneficial properties. The lower caffeine content can also be beneficial, for example, for people with high blood pressure.

Green coffee also contains many antioxidants, which are very important for active people because training can increase the level of oxidation in the body. The presence of oxidants can harm muscles, increase catabolism, and thus limit your athletic capacity and performance.

Black Tea

In the fermentation process of black tea (which lasts longer than other varieties), theaflavins and thearubigins are formed; these compounds have an equally beneficial effect on the body as the antioxidants found in green tea. Black tea is used to alleviate abdominal pain, and with honey and lemon it can relieve some symptoms of a head cold. Black tea's caffeine content ranges from about 25 to 50 milligrams in an 8-ounce cup and depends on the species, the crop, the ripeness of the plant at harvest, and the fermentation method.

Green Tea

Green tea may be the variety most revered for its beneficial effects, particularly because it promotes weight loss, provides many antioxidants, and has some antibacterial properties. Green tea contains iron, zinc, potassium, sodium, and calcium as well as vitamins A, B, B2, B3, B6, C, E, and K.

It is believed that drinking green tea promotes the stabilization of body weight and prevents the accumulation of fatty tissue. Studies on volunteers who for 12 weeks took a green tea extract rich in the antioxidant catechin had a significantly lower body mass and amount of adipose tissue compared to a control group.

Red Tea

A particularly noteworthy variety of red tea is pu-erh (or pu'er). Some studies have shown that this type of tea increases metabolism, resulting in the reduction of body fat. In one research effort, 88 percent of subjects drinking a few cups per day experienced a weight loss of 7–23 pounds while maintaining their current diet. Red tea has been found to support the liver, lower cholesterol, strengthen immunity, and help detoxify the body. It contains many healthy ingredients, such as tannins, alkaloids, flavonoids, minerals (calcium, magnesium, zinc, manganese, copper, selenium), and vitamin C.

White Tea

White tea has been hailed as the elixir of youth because of its polyphenols—a group of antioxidants that fight free radicals. One cup of white tea contains 12 times more polyphenols than a glass of orange juice, which is also considered a rich source of these compounds. White tea also contains ample amounts of vitamin C and caffeine, so it's helpful for people who do intense mental work. The brew from this tea variety is a great alternative to coffee because it is in some ways healthier and it stimulates the body equally well, but it also reduces tension and stress.

CASE STUDY A Runner Optimizes Efficiency with Consistent Hydration

Chris, 16, was a successful runner at the 400m and 800m. He had a basic understanding of sports nutrition, but he struggled to balance his meals on his own, and he also had problems with recovery. His biggest complaints were a lack of energy at track meets, general weakness during training, stomachaches, and dizziness, especially on warm days. It turned out that Chris was not only dehydrated, but he also had an electrolyte imbalance. His troubles were exacerbated by the fact that his coach forbade him to replenish fluids during training, and he prohibited drinking just before the start of important races (the coach allowed just a few sips an hour before competition). According to the coach, drinking 0.5 liter of fluid increased the athlete's body weight by 0.5 kilogram, thus causing poor results on the track.

THE FIX: A loss of even a small amount of fluids (1–2 percent of body weight) disturbs many physiological functions, and it reduces the body's efficiency by up to 10 percent. At any competitive level, a 10 percent drop in efficiency is enormous. Chris was advised to drink 0.5 liter of water about a half an hour before training and track meets. He'd also drink about 0.3 liter of water a few minutes before the first race and an isotonic drink before each subsequent round (for example, before each qualifying heat and the final).

RESULTS: Chris felt much better after the first training session in which he used the new hydration plan. He didn't feel tired, he recovered much faster, and his well-being and motivation improved. He noticed that his workouts began to be more effective, which translated into more success, even at the national level. ■

Alcoholic Beverages

Alcohol is ever present in our world, even among athletes. Long ago, it was credited for improved performance in sports, and it even replaced water in some athletes' mid-race fueling. But alcohol is not beneficial to physical performance. Numerous studies have shown that alcohol does not improve motor skills such as power, strength, speed, and endurance. What's more, after even small amounts of alcohol are consumed, a person's reaction time and ability to concentrate is reduced, and vision can become impaired. About 0.18 grams of alcohol per kilogram of body weight reduces dexterity after 25 minutes: That's one typical 12-ounce beer for a 180-pound male. The American College of Sports Medicine has identified many effects of alcohol that significantly reduce the physical fitness of the body. Alcohol is known to do the following:

> Reduce psychomotor capacity (connection between brain and muscle)
> Cause problems in circulatory and respiratory functions and limit oxygen intake
> Weaken or damage the regulation of body temperature during prolonged exercise, especially in cold environments
> Have a toxic effect on the liver
> Cause hormonal dysfunctions and decrease testosterone concentration in plasma
> Prompt a change in the body's fat metabolism
> Intensify epileptic disorders

Absorption and Digestion of Alcohol

Alcohol is immediately absorbed by the digestive tract and quickly enters all tissues of the body. This happens faster than alcohol can be metabolized. Therefore, its concentration in the blood and tissues initially increases because there is no place in the body where it can be stored, and the only way to reduce its concentration is oxidation. After one drink, the alcohol concentration in the blood reaches peak values in about 40 minutes. This time varies depending on a person's genetic predisposition, the intensity of physical activity, and the presence of other foods in the digestive tract. A small amount (less than 10 percent) can be removed with the urine and through the lungs. Alcohol metabolism takes place in the liver, where it can be oxidized at a rate of 100 milligrams per kilogram of body weight per hour; a person weighing 175 pounds can oxidize 0.8 grams of alcohol per hour. A typical serving of beer or wine has about 14 grams of alcohol.

 Can I have a beer after my run?

Especially among amateur athletes, beer is often celebrated as an ideal post-workout drink. But be careful: There are drawbacks to a beer even though it has benefits, too. Each half liter of beer consumed causes the loss of 700 milliliters of water. The alcohol in beer does not aid in recovery, but the hops and barley are indeed beneficial for the body, so a nonalcoholic beer can be a good post-workout drink. Keep in mind, though, that nonalcoholic beer is not completely free of alcohol: It may contain up to 0.5 percent alcohol.

Beer has a strong antioxidant offering. It contains antioxidant enzymes (for example, catalase, superoxide dismutase, and glutathione peroxidase) and many nonenzymatic compounds with antioxidant effects—mainly phenolic compounds. The hops, depending on the variety, cultivation method, and the conditions for drying and storage, might contain 2–8 percent polyphenols, a group of antioxidants. Other ingredients are beneficial, too. According the United States Department of Agriculture, one can of unpasteurized beer—and many commercial beers are indeed unpasteurized—contains vitamins B1, B2, B3, B6, folic acid, B12, calcium, iron, magnesium, phosphorus, potassium, sodium, and zinc, although not necessarily in high quantity. Pasteurized beer has a lower vitamin and mineral content.

Athletes can afford to have a nonalcoholic beer from time to time after a workout; it will supplement liquids, electrolytes, and vitamins and will fight free radicals, which are abundant after physical activity. You'll likely see beer—nonalcoholic or not—at events like marathons and 5Ks, in fact. They're there, in part, for their beneficial ingredients.

A SNAPSHOT OF ALCOHOL CONSUMPTION IN SPORTS

A study of athletes' drinking habits uncovered trends in professional and amateurs around the world. Among elite Scottish squash players, the consumption of alcohol was about 12 grams per day, providing up to 3 percent of the daily energy demand. (One "standard" 12-ounce beer contains 14 grams of alcohol, as does a 5-ounce glass of wine.) Alcohol consumption was more prevalent in other sports. Australian soccer players consumed 20 grams of alcohol daily, or two standard drinks, according to Australian guidelines.

Alcohol consumption varies among sports. The greatest amount of alcohol consumption is found in soccer, rugby, cricket, football, and golf. About 80 percent of athletes in these sports drink alcohol. Compare those high rates of consumption to other sports: In cycling and tennis, 30 percent consume alcohol.

Nutrition Roundup

The body gradually loses some fluids at rest, and even more during exercise. Follow the guidelines in Table 5.3 to be sure your body is well hydrated for your effort and recovery. Note that after a workout, you should drink more than the amount of body weight lost.

TABLE 5.3 **Your Hydration Plan**

	Timing	Hydration	Other Considerations
Pre-workout >	2 hours before workout	500–600 mL	Include carbs
	30–40 minutes before workout	Okay to drink water	Avoid carbs to prevent a drop in blood sugar at time of workout
After warm-up and before main workout >	If short workout	200–250 mL	Include carbs
	If a prolonged effort (long run/ride)	500–1,000 mL	Include carbs; water volume depends on the weather and other factors
During the workout >	Every 20 minutes	200–300 mL	Short workout: no carbs Long workout: include carbs
Post-workout >	Within 4–6 hours	1,500 mL per kg lost	Include sodium and electrolytes

Weigh yourself before and after your workout to get the most accurate measure of fluids lost.

In fit athletes, sweating during exercise is a good sign, not a bad sign: The body is eliminating excess heat that is generated during exercise. A rise in body temperature can become dangerous; to avoid overheating, the body cools itself by evaporation and other mechanisms. Remaining well hydrated is important to help temperature control.

Losing 1–2 liters of water during exercise disrupts the body's normal functions. Replenishment of fluids both before and during exercise plays an important role in the proper functioning of the body. But too much water may lead to overhydration, which may result in leaching out the sodium that's necessary for the body.

What—and when—you drink matters. The type of fluids consumed should be chosen according to your sport and the duration of the workout, as well as other needs of your body and the weather. Often, water or an electrolyte drink with low carb content is sufficient. Energy drinks and isotonic beverages should not be consumed in excess, and their intake, especially in the case of adolescents, should be under the consultation of a doctor or dietitian.

Tea does not cause dehydration, although this belief has been around for many years (it will dehydrate if one serving contains more than 300 milligrams of caffeine). Tea, which is 99 percent water, contributes to daily hydration needs. Different types of tea have different effects on the body. When choosing a tea, make sure you know what it will do to your body.

Beer will not hydrate your body after an intense workout. Every alcoholic beverage, including beer, dehydrates the body. Nonalcoholic beer does not cause dehydration, though; it has properties similar to an isotonic drink.

Recommended Water Intake

Total daily water consumption depends on your age, sport, training intensity, environment, and local weather. Use the following guidelines but adjust as needed. See the additional recommendations to stay on track of your hydration in Table 5.3.

Body Weight			Daily Water Intake			
(pounds)	(kilograms)		(milliliters)	(liters)	(cups)	(fluid ounces)
100	45	>	1,350	1.35	5.7	45.6
110	50	>	1,500	1.50	6.3	50.7
120	54	>	1,620	1.62	6.8	54.8
130	59	>	1,770	1.77	7.5	59.9
140	64	>	1,920	1.92	8.1	64.9
150	68	>	2,040	2.04	8.6	69.0
160	73	>	2,190	2.19	9.3	74.1
170	77	>	2,310	2.31	9.8	78.1
180	82	>	2,460	2.46	10.4	83.2
190	86	>	2,580	2.58	10.9	87.2
200	91	>	2,730	2.73	11.5	92.3
210	95	>	2,850	2.85	12.0	96.4
220	100	>	3,000	3.00	12.7	101.4

Continues

Continued

Body Weight			Daily Water Intake			
(pounds)	(kilograms)		(milliliters)	(liters)	(cups)	(fluid ounces)
230	104	>	3,120	3.12	13.2	105.5
240	109	>	3,270	3.27	13.8	110.6
250	113	>	3,390	3.39	14.3	114.6
260	118	>	3,540	3.54	15.0	119.7
270	122	>	3,660	3.66	15.5	123.8
280	127	>	3,810	3.81	16.1	128.8
290	132	>	3,960	3.96	16.7	133.9
300	136	>	4,080	4.08	17.2	138.0

Note: Calculations assume a recommendation of drinking 30 milliliters of water for every kilogram of body weight. Excludes hydration needs during and after exercise.

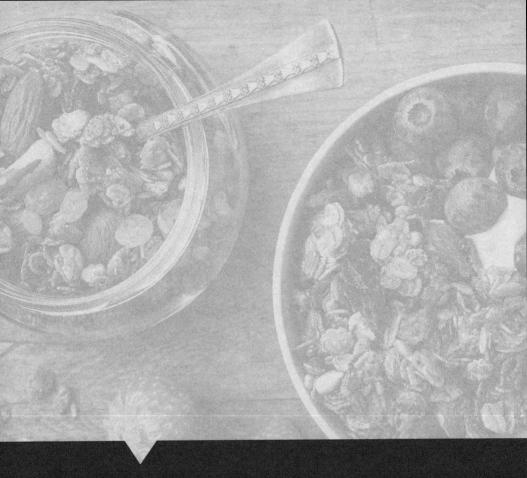

6 | SAMPLE MEAL PLANS

Now that you have learned how your body uses food to fuel your sport, let's see what a full day of well-planned nutrition would look like. The following sample meal plans were designed for athletes participating in strength training, swimming, cycling, martial arts, soccer, and running. A ketogenic diet is also detailed. These meal plans demonstrate the concepts explained throughout earlier chapters: adequate fueling before and during a workout, consistent hydration, well-timed recovery, and an emphasis on nutrient- and vitamin-rich, high-quality foods.

These diets don't apply only to the particular sports listed, though; if you participate in a different sport, choose the diet for a sport that has similar energy and training requirements. And be sure to review the other diets to grow your repertoire of go-to meals and snacks. (Chapter 7, "Recipes," presents more meals with complete preparation instructions.)

The meals below are suggestions; feel free to adapt them to your preferences and availability of ingredients. Note that the total calories provided by these diets are suitable for moderately to highly active people training consistently throughout the week; be sure to adapt or reduce the caloric intake on rest days or during less busy seasons.

Strength Training and Bodybuilding

For a lean person to gain a bodybuilder's physique, training and adequate nutrition are extremely important. Proteins are the primary building block for muscle growth, but eating too much protein (more than 2 grams per kilogram of body weight) will not cause faster muscle growth, as this excess will be excreted in the urine and not retained and converted into muscle. There are periods when you can afford such a high amount of protein, however, but only for a few weeks of very intense training at a time, not throughout the entire year.

Protein is found in both animal and plant sources. The ratio between animal and vegetable proteins should be 3 to 1. Plants are a source of not only valuable amino acids, but also fiber, which helps move fecal matter and neutralize putrefaction, a form of decomposition that often arises in the intestines as a result of the consumption of large amounts of protein.

Carbohydrates also play a very important role in strength training, and those that slowly release energy are the most desirable. Foods that provide such low- or medium-GI carbs include oatmeal, buckwheat, brown pasta, multigrain bread, and brown rice.

The amount of protein recommended for strength sports ranges from 1.2 to 2.0 grams per kilogram of body weight per day (0.54–0.9 g/lb). Carbohydrates are important whether the bodybuilder is working on trimming down, muscle definition, or muscle growth. Generally, on nontraining days the amount of carbohydrates should be 3–5 grams per kilogram of body weight per day (1.36–2.27 g/lb), and on training days, 5–8 grams per kilogram of body weight per day (2.27–3.64 g/lb). However, as mentioned before, the actual amount needed depends on the purpose of the training, performance level, sex, metabolic efficiency, and more. You should also not completely exclude fats from your diet. Healthy fats are very important, even in such disciplines as bodybuilding, general fitness, powerlifting, or weight lifting. Consider healthy sources of unsaturated fats—for example, peanut butter or pumpkin and sunflower seeds.

In an athlete with a high metabolism, acquiring energy and nutrients from food may not be enough during periods of intense training. In this case, supplements become an indispensable part of the daily diet. To support protein intake, focus on supplementing with a variety of proteins, depending on the time of day. The most important is casein, which, taken later in the day, can limit catabolic processes during sleep. Some athletes choose to eat a nearly exclusively protein-based dinner, which is somewhat justified: It accelerates nocturnal regeneration and does not cause an increase in body fat. In addition, carbohydrate consumption in the evening contributes to the secretion of insulin, which blocks the release of growth hormone. On the other hand, an athlete who cannot easily increase body weight should not go without carbohydrates in the evening. These energy sources, consumed in sufficient amounts during the day and evening, cause the accumulation of muscle glycogen, which gives more volume to the muscles. Any carbohydrates eaten later in the day should be complex carbs so that they do not cause rapid secretion of insulin, which—as you know—may promote the deposition of fat.

Athletes in strength sports often prepare very simple meals, such as rice with chicken and vegetables or oatmeal cooked with water. Their diets are also sometimes augmented with excessive amounts of protein supplements. Fruits provide antioxidants, and yogurt acts as a protein source. If you are lactose intolerant, you can seek out Greek yogurt with a lower carbohydrate content (and therefore lower lactose content—depending on your level of sensitivity). In order to maintain the feeling of satiety for a longer time, add some healthy fats in the form of almonds; these can be replaced by walnuts or hazelnuts.

To add variety to your diet, consider replacing rice with other grains, such as the farro, buckwheat, and barley used in these meals. And experiment with meats that have high biological value; chicken and beef don't need to be the only options.

Beets are included because they are a good source of folic acid and the antioxidant betanin. To preserve more of their flavor and nutrients, bake them whole and then peel them (or rub the skins off using a rag or towel that you don't mind turning red), to lose as little of their flavor and nutritional value as possible. To lower their glycemic load, you can drizzle some olive oil on them.

When building muscle mass, your diet should be full of wholesome protein, preferably in every meal and certainly in the meal after your workout. To fuel hard workouts in the gym, an adequate supply of carbohydrates is just as important as the protein that then builds muscle. Sometimes, inexperienced athletes hope muscle gains will come simply by eating a high-protein diet and working out a little, but there's more to it than that. For muscles to increase in size, they need to experience damage at the fiber level. Then, proper regeneration is essential. Strength training every day, with no recovery periods, will not bring you the desired results because the regeneration period (overnight) is too short. Large muscle groups need up to four days to recover and rebuild from the stress of training. And, of course, they need proper nutrition.

If it is difficult to cover the demand for carbohydrates with rice or whole grains, dried fruits are a good addition. Eat them in moderation, though, because most have a moderate to high glycemic index. And with their higher

Strength Training and Bodybuilding

The following sample diet was designed to increase muscle mass for a 28-year-old man in strength sports. He weighs 190 pounds, is 6'2", and trains in the evening on most days of the week.

1 YOGURT WITH BARLEY, FRUIT, AND ALMONDS

	Serving		Energy (cal)	Protein (g)	Fat (g)	Carbs (g)
Pearled barley flakes	1 cup	>	408	11.5	1.3	72
Strawberries	1 cup	>	44.8	1	0.6	10.1
Almonds	2 Tbsp	>	85.8	3	7.8	3.1
Natural yogurt, 2% fat	1 cup	>	155	12.9	3.8	17
Banana	1 medium	>	116.4	1.2	0.4	28.2
TOTAL		>	810	29.6	13.9	130.4

2 TUNA PATTIES

	Serving		Energy (cal)	Protein (g)	Fat (g)	Carbs (g)
Buckwheat flour	1 cup	>	300	10	1	62
Tomato	1 large	>	32.6	1.7	0.4	6.9
Tuna in water, drained	3 oz	>	95	21	1.2	0
Onion	¼ medium	>	11.6	0.5	0.1	2.4
Canola oil	1 tsp	>	45	0	5	0
Parsley	1 Tbsp	>	2	0.2	0	0.4
Black pepper	1 tsp	>	2.5	0.1	0	0.6
TOTAL		>	488.7	33.5	7.7	72.3

3 CHICKEN AND VEGGIE WRAPS

	Serving	Energy (cal)	Protein (g)	Fat (g)	Carbs (g)
Whole-grain tortilla	Two 6-inch	194.1	5.4	4.3	32.5
Avocado	½ medium	113	1.3	10.5	5.9
Lettuce, chopped	½ cup	5	0.3	0	1
Cherry tomatoes, fresh	½ cup chopped	15	0.9	0.2	3.6
Meat from chicken or turkey drumsticks, without skin	1 oz	50	8.3	1.9	0
Cream cheese	1 Tbsp	50	0.9	5	0.25
Dried tomatoes in olive oil	1 Tbsp	15	0.35	1	1.6
TOTAL		442.1	17.45	22.9	44.85

4 PORK TENDERLOIN WITH FARRO AND BEETS

	Serving	Energy (cal)	Protein (g)	Fat (g)	Carbs (g)
Farro, cooked	½ cup	280	12	0	60
Roasted pork tenderloin	5 oz	202	37.1	5	0
Beets, cubed	1 cup	75	2.9	0	16.9
Canola oil	1 Tbsp	120	0	13.6	0
TOTAL		677	52	18.6	76.9

5 FRUIT AND ALMOND SMOOTHIE

	Serving	Energy (cal)	Protein (g)	Fat (g)	Carbs (g)
Almond butter	1 Tbsp	98	3.3	8.9	3
Banana	1 medium	105	1.3	0.4	27
Blackberries	1 cup	62	2	0.7	13.8
Millet flakes	½ cup	220	6	3	46
TOTAL		485	12.6	13	89.8

POST-WORKOUT PROTEIN DRINK & APRICOTS AND TURKEY WITH VEGETABLES

	Serving	Energy (cal)	Protein (g)	Fat (g)	Carbs (g)
Recovery drink	2 scoops (~75 g)	280	27	2.5	38
Apricots, dried	¼ cup	100	1	0	26
Turkey breast meat, without skin	3 oz	108	22.9	1.8	0
Asparagus	10 medium spears	33	3.6	0.3	6.2
Yogurt, 2% fat	⅓ cup	27.8	2.2	0.8	3.1
Red bell pepper, chopped	½ cup	23	0.7	0.2	4.5
Canola oil	1 Tbsp	63	0	7	0
Fresh mushrooms, sliced	½ cup	8	1.1	0.1	1.1
Brown rice, cooked	⅔ cup	166	3.7	1.3	34.5
TOTAL		808.8	62.2	14	113.4

STRENGTH TRAINING AND BODYBUILDING DAILY TOTAL

Meal		Energy (cal)	Protein (g)	Fat (g)	Carbs (g)
1	>	810	29.6	13.9	130.4
2	>	488.7	33.5	7.7	72.3
3	>	442.1	17.45	22.9	44.85
4	>	677	52	18.6	76.9
5	>	485	12.6	13	89.8
6	>	808.8	62.2	14	113.4
TOTAL	>	3,711.60	207.35	90.1	527.65

concentration of fiber, they're not recommended immediately before training. But at other times of the day, a good option is dried apricots, which have a low glycemic index (30) and are one of the better sources of lycopene, a powerful antioxidant. Due to their large supply of base-forming constituents, dried apricots are recommended for hyperacidity of the stomach and at times when the body is more acidic, such as after physical exertion. Try to find dried, unsulfured apricots; they'll have a brown color, while yellow or orange dried apricots will likely be sulfured, meaning they have been preserved with sulfur dioxide.

During times of heavy training loads (four to five workouts per week with heavy weights) the amount of carbohydrates needed after training can reach up to 1.5–2 grams per kilogram of body weight to fully compensate for the loss of glycogen. This amount should be divided into two or three portions within the first two hours after your workout. It is best to first eat carbohydrates that are absorbed quickly (those with a high glycemic index), while subsequent meals should provide carbohydrates with medium and low GI values to avoid spikes in insulin.

Cycling

Nutrition plans in endurance sports should be based on a sufficiently large quantity of carbohydrates because they are a primary source of energy, especially in the first half hour of effort. It is assumed that the muscles of athletes practicing endurance sports use about 1 gram of glucose per minute of effort. For long, intense training, even 10 grams of carbohydrates per kilogram of body weight is recommended (some riders racing in the Tour de France consume even 14 grams per kilogram of body weight each day). Numerous scientific studies show that athletes training for two to three hours, five or six days per week, should have a carbohydrate intake of 5–8 grams per kilograms of body weight per day, or 2.27–3.64 grams per pound.

Remember that if training or a race lasts longer than 90 minutes, you can consume 30–60 grams of carbs per hour; if the weather is cold, the amount may be even higher to protect your body heat.

Carbohydrates can limit the damaging process of catabolism. During very long and intense efforts, the body begins to generate energy from the amino acids accumulated in muscles, which leads to the destruction of those muscles. What follows is the intensified production of ammonia and urea, which accelerates dehydration. Numerous studies have demonstrated that the intake of carbohydrates during extremely long efforts significantly reduces the release of ammonia and urea and thus reduces muscle catabolism. Less muscle fatigue also reduces the time needed for regeneration, allowing you to get back on the bike sooner.

We also shouldn't underestimate the role of fats in cycling, as they are an important source of energy, and with longer efforts of low or medium intensity, fats will have a larger role in supplying energy. The ability to use fats for energy increases as the athlete's fitness improves. In well-trained cyclists, fats can provide up to 44 percent of energy when cycling with an intensity of 50 percent VO_2max (maximum oxygen uptake). In contrast, untrained people would receive just 33 percent of their energy from fat oxidation during the same effort. Cycling is, therefore, a good sport to take up if you want to reduce body fat—assuming your efforts stay within the fat-burning heart rate ranges.

Cycling also requires a substantial supply of protein, which sometimes reaches 2 grams per kilogram of body weight or more, although most recommendations range from 1.2 to 2.0 grams per kilogram. It's beneficial to combine carbohydrates with protein. In research conducted on cyclists, taking a carbohydrate-protein solution every 20 minutes during several hours of effort delayed the onset of fatigue by 14 minutes, while in the group receiving only carbohydrates, the time was half as long.

Other studies have shown that the intake of carbohydrates along with protein significantly improves the regeneration of energy reserves after the workout. The study was performed on trained cyclists who took a drink containing protein (28 grams) and sugars (106 grams) immediately after a two-hour training ride and again two hours later. Their resistance to fatigue was 55 percent greater compared to a group that only took a carbohydrate drink (42 grams). The combination of carbohydrates and protein can significantly

Cycling

The following early-season diet was developed for a 23-year-old male cyclist weighing 175 pounds, training in the evenings.

1   QUINOA BREAKFAST BOWL WITH FRUIT

	Serving	Energy (cal)	Protein (g)	Fat (g)	Carbs (g)
Quinoa, cooked	1 cup	220	8.1	3.6	39.4
Cocoa	1 Tbsp	23	0.9	1.1	2.5
Banana	1 medium	116.4	1.2	0.4	28.2
Medjool dates	2 each	110	1	0	31
Almond butter	2 Tbsp	196	6.7	7.7	6
Unsweetened rice milk	1 cup	70	0	2.5	11
TOTAL		735.4	17.9	15.3	118.1

2   RYE TOAST WITH CAMEMBERT & ARUGULA AND A MIXED VEGGIE DRINK

	Serving	Energy (cal)	Protein (g)	Fat (g)	Carbs (g)
Rye bread	2 slices	165	5.4	2.1	30.9
Butter	1 Tbsp	102	0.1	11.5	0.1
Camembert cheese	2 oz	170	11.2	13.8	0.2
Arugula	½ cup	2.5	0.2	0	0.4
Multi-vegetable juice	1 cup	53	1.5	0.2	11.1
TOTAL		492.5	18.4	27.6	42.7

3   SHRIMP STIR-FRY

	Serving	Energy (cal)	Protein (g)	Fat (g)	Carbs (g)
Rice noodles	2 cups, cooked	380	6.3	0.7	84.5
Zucchini, sliced	2 cups	54	4.1	1.3	9.7
Sesame seeds	2 Tbsp	103	3.2	8.9	4.2
Frozen shrimp, thawed	4 oz	112	27.2	0.3	0.2
TOTAL		649	40.8	11.2	98.6

4   SPICED COCONUT AND COFFEE SMOOTHIE

	Serving	Energy (cal)	Protein (g)	Fat (g)	Carbs (g)
Espresso coffee	2.5 oz	6.3	0.1	0.1	1.2
Coconut milk, canned	½ cup	223	2.3	24.2	3.2
Banana	1 medium	116.4	1.2	0.4	28.2
Medjool dates	2 each	110	1	0	31
Cocoa	1 Tbsp	23	0.9	1.1	2.5
Turmeric powder	1 tsp	6.8	0.2	0.7	1.5
Cardamom	½ tsp	3.1	0.1	0.1	0.7
TOTAL		488.6	7.8	26.6	68.3

5   MID-RIDE AND POST-WORKOUT SNACKS

	Serving	Energy (cal)	Protein (g)	Fat (g)	Carbs (g)
Sports drink (mid-ride)	25 oz	217.5	0	0	50.3
Sports drink	16 oz	120	1	0	28
Medjool dates	2 each	110	1	0	31
Protein bar	1 each	190	20	8	5
TOTAL		637.5	22	8	114.3

6   COD WITH COUSCOUS AND VEGETABLES

	Serving	Energy (cal)	Protein (g)	Fat (g)	Carbs (g)
Baked Cod	4 oz >	120	25.9	1	0
Couscous	½ cup, dry >	333	12.1	1.5	69.7
Zucchini, sliced	2 cups >	38.3	2.7	0.2	7.2
Crushed tomatoes, canned	½ cup >	40	2	0	6
Red bell pepper, chopped	½ cup >	23	0.7	0.2	4.5
Onion	½ medium >	22.5	0.5	0.3	6
Garlic	1 clove >	9.1	0.4	0	2
TOTAL	>	585.9	44.3	3.2	95.4

CYCLING DAILY TOTAL

Meal	Energy (cal)	Protein (g)	Fat (g)	Carbs (g)
1 >	735.4	17.9	15.3	118.1
2 >	492.5	18.4	27.6	42.7
3 >	649	40.8	11.2	98.6
4 >	488.6	7.8	26.6	68.3
5 >	637.5	22	8	114.3
6 >	585.9	44.3	3.2	95.4
TOTAL >	3,588.9	151.2	91.9	537.4

improve the body's regenerative efforts: catabolic processes associated with a long-term endurance effort can be reduced by up to 83 percent.

The proposed menu includes quinoa because it is a great alternative to the popular oatmeal. Quinoa contains all the essential amino acids, is gluten-free, and falls on the low end of the glycemic index. In addition, it is a good source of magnesium, potassium, B vitamins, folic acid, and fiber. It is a powerful grain and a great staple for the active person.

A good add-in for oatmeal, sandwiches, or smoothies is high-quality nut butter, which slows energy release from carbohydrates due to its healthy fats. There is a difference between butter from peanuts, which is a legume, and true nuts like walnuts and almonds; the latter contain healthy fats, vitamin E, and a good helping of magnesium.

Each meal in this sample plan contains carbohydrates that allow you to build up the right amount of glycogen for a long workout. In addition, protein from animals will not generally need to surpass 35–45 grams per serving. The situation is slightly different in the case of vegetable protein: Due to the incomplete share of essential amino acids, its value counts as about 50 percent of the quantity eaten (this difference between plant and animal proteins is explained in Chapter 3). In other words, if you eat 50 grams of incomplete vegetable protein, you count half of it—25 grams—as a wholesome protein in the diet.

A meal after training should contain at least 1 gram of carbohydrates per kilogram of body weight.

Swimming

An effective nutrition plan in a discipline such as swimming, especially in adolescents, is extremely important. This is mainly due to training patterns in swimming: Often, swimmers have two or even three sessions per day. With an early-morning session, it's important for a swimmer to fuel properly not only for that first session, but to start the day off right for fueling in subsequent hours. In the early morning, if it's not possible to eat a full meal in advance of the workout, a liquid or semiliquid breakfast or an appropriate supplement can guard the body against hypoglycemia. The lack of breakfast slows down metabolism because after a night of hunger, the body needs a new dose of energy, and if it does not get one, it begins to reserve resources and slow down processes in the body. In the long term, this leads to fat deposition and a lack of energy when the athlete needs it most.

The daily energy expenditure of an adult swimmer varies between 3,600 and 6,100 calories depending on age, sex, training load, style, and swimming speed. Numerous researchers determined that the total energy expenditure of swimmers covering an average distance of 9 kilometers per day was about 4,600 calories.

During workouts at an intensity of 65–85 percent VO_2max, the main factor limiting an athlete's exercise capacity is the amount of muscle glycogen available. Studies show that swimmers will have lost 12 percent of their glycogen after an interval workout. To rebuild these resources within 24 hours after the effort, the right amount of carbohydrates in the diet is important. Carbohydrates should contribute 65 percent or even 70 percent of a swimmer's caloric intake; for a 4,600-calorie diet, that equates to 750–805 grams of carbohydrates per day.

Poor nutrition, especially in teenaged swimmers, may impair their physical and mental development, weaken the immune system, and increase the incidence of infectious diseases. An unbalanced diet will also impede a swimmer's performance, leading to overtraining and possibly injury.

This swimmer's menu was primarily aimed at a slight caloric restriction during a specific training block. Breakfast in the form of a smoothie is a good option before entering the water. It is not too high in calories, and because the morning training mostly stays within the aerobic zone, there isn't as great a demand for carbs. As this swimmer was trying to lose a little weight, the morning session is helpful because it remains aerobic and thereby encourages the body to generate energy from adipose tissue.

Smoothies made with yogurt or kefir make healthy morning meals for a swimmer; athletes with lactose intolerance could use lactose-free milk or

Swimming

Below is a sample day from the diet of a 17-year-old male swimmer. His goal was to reduce body fat by 3–4 percent; he weighs 138 pounds. The swimmer participates in two training sessions per day: 45 minutes in the morning and 90 minutes in the afternoon.

1 MANGO SMOOTHIE

	Serving		Energy (cal)	Protein (g)	Fat (g)	Carbs (g)
Soy milk	1 cup	>	90	6.5	3	9.3
Mango, cubed	1 cup	>	82.8	0.6	0.4	20.4
Almond butter	1¼ Tbsp	>	122.8	4.2	11.1	3.8
TOTAL		>	295.6	11.3	14.5	33.5

2 POST-WORKOUT BREAKFAST

	Serving		Energy (cal)	Protein (g)	Fat (g)	Carbs (g)
Sports drink	16 oz	>	145	0	0	33.5
Diced peaches, canned in juice	1 cup	>	109	1.6	0.1	28.7
Cottage cheese, low-fat	1 cup	>	160	28	1	6
Baby carrots	10 each	>	35	0.6	0	8.2
Vegetable juice	1 cup	>	51	2	0	10
TOTAL		>	500	30.2	1.1	86.4

3   SALMON SALAD WITH QUINOA AND GRAPEFRUIT

	Serving		Energy (cal)	Protein (g)	Fat (g)	Carbs (g)
Smoked salmon	3 oz	>	99.5	15.6	3.7	0
Grapefruit	½ medium	>	60	1	0	15
Romaine lettuce, chopped	2 cups	>	20	1.3	0	4
Pecans, chopped	2 Tbsp	>	94.2	1.3	9.8	1.9
Quinoa, cooked	1 cup	>	222	8.1	3.6	39.4
TOTAL		>	495.7	27.3	17.1	60.3

4   SPAGHETTI WITH TURKEY, SPINACH, AND SUN-DRIED TOMATOES

	Serving		Energy (cal)	Protein (g)	Fat (g)	Carbs (g)
Whole-wheat spaghetti, cooked	1 cup	>	174	7	2	35.2
Spinach, fresh	1 cup	>	13.3	1.3	0	2
Skinless turkey breast	3 oz	>	125	25.6	1.8	0
Sun-dried tomatoes	1 Tbsp	>	8.7	0.5	0.1	1.9
Garlic	1 clove	>	4.5	0.2	0	1
Canola oil	1 Tbsp	>	123.8	0	14	0
TOTAL		>	449.6	34.6	17.9	40.1

5   PRE-WORKOUT SNACK

	Serving		Energy (cal)	Protein (g)	Fat (g)	Carbs (g)
Sports drink	16 oz	>	145	0	0	33.5
Banana	1 medium	>	116.4	1.2	0.4	28.2
TOTAL		>	261.4	1.2	0.4	61.7

6 CHICKEN AND VEGETABLE SKEWERS

	Serving		Energy (cal)	Protein (g)	Fat (g)	Carbs (g)
Skinless chicken breast, roasted	3 oz	>	128.4	26	2.7	0
Red bell pepper, chopped	1 cup	>	46.2	1.5	0.5	9
Cherry tomatoes, chopped	½ cup	>	15	1	0.2	3
Onion	1 medium	>	44	1.2	0.1	10.3
Fresh mushrooms, sliced	1 cup	>	21.1	3	0.3	3.1
Curry seasoning	1 tsp	>	0	0	0	0
TOTAL		>	254.7	32.7	3.8	25.4

SWIMMING DAILY TOTAL

Meal		Energy (cal)	Protein (g)	Fat (g)	Carbs (g)
1	>	295.6	11.3	14.5	33.5
2	>	500	30.2	1.1	86.4
3	>	495.7	27.3	17.1	60.3
4	>	449.6	34.6	17.9	40.1
5	>	261.4	1.2	0.4	61.7
6	>	254.7	32.7	3.8	25.4
TOTAL	>	2,257	137.3	54.8	307.4

coconut water. Add a small amount of healthy fats—for example, avocado—and chia seeds, berries, and millet flakes. Dairy-based snacks or meals are also beneficial as part of the daily diet because they are a valuable source of calcium necessary to build and maintain proper bone density. And a study conducted on more than 10,000 people showed the inverse correlation between calcium intake and body mass: More calcium in the diet correlated with lower body weight.

Dairy products have a beneficial effect on body weight because of their calcium and whey protein content. Intracellular calcium concentration is an important factor regulating the metabolism of adipocytes (fat cells), affecting how they utilize and store triglycerides. High calcium intake will therefore contribute to the inhibition of fatty acid synthesis and an increase in lipolysis, which in turn leads to the reduction of adipose tissue. In addition, increased calcium intake is accompanied by increased fat excretion in the feces, so the calories available to the body are reduced. Numerous studies also report that dairy products reduce visceral fat.

Yogurts are a good base for morning smoothies, even for people with lactose intolerance, because through fermentation and the presence of bacterial strains, gastric problems are in most cases minimized or nonexistent. However, if gastric problems occur, you can exclude dairy, using calcium-enriched lactose-free products or plant substitutes (for example, rice, almond, or soy milk) instead.

The post-workout meal provides foods that release carbs quickly (through the isotonic sports drink) and slowly (the carbohydrates in cottage cheese) to rebuild lost glycogen reserves. This refueling is important because although the body derived a lot of energy from fat, glycogen was also depleted. The body needs sufficient refueling, especially because another training session—the more intense workout—will start in less than 12 hours. Foods rich in protein help rebuild microtears in the muscles, and vegetables provide antioxidants to further promote recovery. Additionally, an adequate level of hydration is important so as not to interfere with metabolic and physiological processes by lowering fluid levels.

Martial Arts

Martial arts, such as boxing, jiujitsu, or kickboxing, require exceptional endurance and strength, but they also demand great resistance to injuries and very efficient regeneration. Competition usually takes place at high intensity, sometimes lasting up to half an hour. Athletes remain in almost constant muscle tension and must be extremely focused from the first to the last second, which places a great demand on the nervous system. All of this means that martial artists' energy consumption is high, so taking care of the diet is of particular importance here. The specific discipline influences the caloric demand; for example, boxing matches may last 36 minutes, and jiujitsu matches last 5–10 minutes. In general, though, an athlete's caloric intake might range from 2,800 to 4,200 calories. The athlete's performance level and the amount of training is also a factor.

The athlete's weight, which in some of these sports is strictly regulated, also affects diet choices. This places more importance on proper nutrition, both during the preparatory period and in the final phase of adjusting to a goal weight before a competition. Often, athletes aim to lose several pounds (in extreme cases, up to 20 pounds) within a few days or weeks. Early in their preparatory period, they work on strength, power, and general conditioning, so they might not follow a diet as closely, and consequently they may gain a few extra pounds. Quick weight loss in the final days before a match is never beneficial because the weight likely comes from rapid dehydration and glycogen depletion—neither of which is helpful—and not body fat. Losing a pound or less the day before a match is different from trying to get rid of several pounds over a week. The latter could be avoided if the competitor ate sensibly a few weeks before the fight to avoid extra fat deposition.

In martial arts, the training plan quite often includes two sessions per day. In the case of this athlete, morning workouts stayed in the aerobic zone to reduce body fat. Although more fat was used for energy in this workout, the muscles still experienced some damage, so regeneration must be fast, in time for the afternoon session. The second workout usually involves exercises,

Martial Arts

The following sample meal plan was developed for a 172-pound athlete who performs aerobic training in the morning and a mat workout in the afternoon.

1 PRE-WORKOUT SNACK

	Serving		Energy (cal)	Protein (g)	Fat (g)	Carbs (g)
Rice cakes, apple cinnamon flavor	2 each	>	100	2	0	22
Almond butter	2 Tbsp	>	196	6.7	17.8	6
TOTAL		>	296	8.7	17.8	28

2 RECOVERY DRINK AND A FRUIT SMOOTHIE

	Serving		Energy (cal)	Protein (g)	Fat (g)	Carbs (g)
Sports drink	16 oz	>	145	0	0	33.5
Medjool dates	2 each	>	110	1	0	31
Whey protein isolate	~1 scoop	>	71.9	17.6	0.1	0.1
Quinoa, cooked	⅔ cup	>	73.6	2.8	1.2	12.8
Banana	1 medium	>	105	1.3	0.4	27
Raspberries	1 cup	>	63	1.5	0.8	14.7
Milk, 1% fat	1 cup	>	102	8.2	2.4	12.1
TOTAL		>	670.5	32.4	4.9	131.2

3   VEGETABLE SALAD WITH MILLET AND FETA CHEESE

	Serving		Energy (cal)	Protein (g)	Fat (g)	Carbs (g)
Spinach	1 cup	>	13.3	1.3	0	2
Feta cheese	¼ cup	>	99	5.3	8	1.5
Zucchini, sliced	2 cups	>	38.4	2.7	0.7	7
Fresh parsley, chopped	2 Tbsp	>	2.7	0.2	0	0.4
Mustard	1 Tbsp	>	9	0.6	0.5	0.9
Olive oil	1 Tbsp	>	119	0	13.5	0
Lemon juice	1 Tbsp	>	3	0	1	0
Millet, cooked	1 cup	>	207	6.1	1.7	41.1
Red bell peppers, chopped	1 cup	>	46.2	1.5	0.5	9
TOTAL		>	537.6	17.7	25.9	61.9

4   CHICKEN WITH RICE AND VEGETABLES

	Serving		Energy (cal)	Protein (g)	Fat (g)	Carbs (g)
Skinless chicken breast, roasted	3 oz	>	128.4	26	2.7	0
Red bell pepper, chopped	1 cup	>	46.2	1.5	0.5	9
Cherry tomatoes, chopped	½ cup	>	15	1	0.2	3
Onion	1 medium	>	44	1.2	0.1	10.3
Fresh mushrooms, sliced	1 cup	>	21.1	3	0.3	3.1
Canola oil	1 Tbsp	>	123.7	0	14	0
Garlic	1 clove	>	9.1	0.4	0	2
Brown rice, cooked	1 cup	>	248.5	5.5	1.9	51.7
TOTAL		>	636	38.6	19.7	79.1

5 POST-WORKOUT SNACK

	Serving	Energy (cal)	Protein (g)	Fat (g)	Carbs (g)
Sports drink	~25 oz	> 217.5	0	0	50.3
Protein bar	1 each	> 304.8	23.7	10.6	33
TOTAL		> 522.3	23.7	10.6	83.3

6 SPICY PASTA AND SHRIMP

	Serving	Energy (cal)	Protein (g)	Fat (g)	Carbs (g)
Rice noodles, cooked	1 cup	> 190	3.1	0.3	42.2
Cooked shrimp	3 oz	> 84.2	20.4	0.2	0.2
Red chili peppers, chopped	4 Tbsp	> 12	0.6	0.1	2.6
Fresh cilantro	1 Tbsp	> 0.7	0.1	0	0.1
Fresh basil	1 Tbsp	> 0.7	0.1	0	0.1
Parmesan cheese	1 Tbsp	> 21.6	1.9	1.4	0.2
Clarified butter	1 tsp	> 44.1	0	5	0
TOTAL		> 353.3	26.2	7	45.4

MARTIAL ARTS DAILY TOTAL

Meal	Energy (cal)	Protein (g)	Fat (g)	Carbs (g)
1 >	296	8.7	17.8	28
2 >	670.5	32.4	4.9	131.2
3 >	537.6	17.7	25.9	61.9
4 >	636	38.6	19.7	79.1
5 >	522.3	23.7	10.6	83.3
6 >	353.3	26.2	7	45.4
TOTAL >	3,015.70	147.3	85.9	428.9

including intervals, that reach higher heart rates, so carbohydrates before and after training is an essential element of a proper diet.

Don't wait too long to eat a meal after training because the sooner you start refueling, the faster and more effective the body's recuperation will be. Try to eat a meal in a liquid or semiliquid form within 20–30 minutes after the workout, and remember to drink water, too. After an effort, the body needs 5–10 minutes for all systems (including circulatory and respiratory systems) to cool down to a resting state; then the absorption of nutrients will be easier.

There are frequent meals in this plan to gradually deliver carbohydrates and thus accumulate energy for the afternoon workout without straining the digestive system. To this end, most carbohydrates in this meal plan have low or medium glycemic index values. The banana, in particular, can be used strategically to manage carbs. For pre-workout snacking, an unripe banana (one with a green peel) is helpful, while immediately after training, a really ripe banana with some browning on the peel is more appropriate. Green bananas contain more starch and less water compared to very ripe, brown bananas, and they have a medium glycemic index. On the other hand, ripe bananas quickly release energy, which is why they are ideal for glycogen resynthesis. Bananas are not only a source of energy, but also of potassium and antioxidative vitamins such as A, C, and E.

Dates also work well as a supplement to carbohydrates, which is why they are included. They replenish glycogen and provide a healthy serving of potassium, one of the electrolytes lost through sweat.

The last meal of the day contains small amounts of carbohydrates in order to gradually restore glycogen, a wholesome protein, and healthy fats to prolong the release of substrates necessary for regeneration. In some cases, especially for people with some extra body fat, carbohydrates can be removed from the last meal, but then to feel more full and satiated, consider adding fatty fish (for example, salmon or mackerel) in combination with vegetables.

Forgoing carbs at dinner, to help with fat loss, is only possible because the post-workout snack (meal 5) provides adequate amounts of carbs. So the body is refueled then, and the dinner can focus on protein and fat. These will regenerate muscles and support anticatabolic activity. Fats will extend this process of protecting the muscles during sleep. Fats could come from sunflower seeds, pumpkin seeds, or nuts.

Soccer

Soccer players cover an average of 4–7 miles during a game: 24 percent of the game is spent is walking, 36 percent jogging, 20 percent running, and 11 percent sprinting. Players in the Champions League often cover more than 9 miles. To have sufficient energy for a big game that includes plenty of high-end efforts, it is necessary to have a proper diet.

A soccer player who trains twice daily needs a regular intake of carbohydrates throughout the day for both recovery and fueling for the next workout. To help the body extract energy from carbohydrates and building blocks from proteins, B-group vitamins are crucial. Whole-grain cereals offer these and other valuable vitamins and micronutrients. For variety and high nutrient content, consider using grain flakes from unroasted groats, which, unlike roasted grains, have many more nutrients and a more delicate flavor. In addition, this type of groats alkalizes the body, so it is worth using in the diet to maintain a proper acid-base balance.

The many intense efforts in soccer can lead to an increased production of oxygen free radicals in skeletal muscles, blood, and other tissues. This diet includes goji berries, besides other fresh fruits and vegetables, to help reduce the presence of these damaging compounds. Dried and ripe fruits are often rich in vitamin C. It is estimated that 100 grams of berries contain up to 2,500 milligrams of this vitamin, which puts the goji fruit in third place among natural sources of vitamin C. Note that no more than 30–40 berries should be eaten every day; this portion provides about 500 milligrams of vitamin C, which is enough for a single serving—and the body will not absorb any more of it. Moreover, larger amounts of goji berries may cause stomach problems. Long-term use of goji berries has been connected to improved immunity and joint and bone health, and it has a positive effect on vision.

Soccer

This diet was created for a 26-year-old soccer player who trains twice daily: general development and team tactics 10:00 a.m. to 11:00 a.m. and full-field practice 4:00 p.m. to 6:00 p.m.

1   WHOLE-GRAIN CEREAL WITH FRUIT

	Serving		Energy (cal)	Protein (g)	Fat (g)	Carbs (g)
Strawberries, sliced	1 cup	>	48	1	0.6	10.8
Goji berries	2½ Tbsp	>	55.8	2.3	0.1	12.3
Wheat flakes cereal	2 cups	>	252	7.8	1.9	63.1
Walnuts, chopped	3 Tbsp	>	133.2	3.2	12.1	3.6
TOTAL		>	489	14.3	14.7	89.8

2   BLUEBERRY AND SPINACH SMOOTHIE

	Serving		Energy (cal)	Protein (g)	Fat (g)	Carbs (g)
Coconut water	~25 oz	>	142.5	5.2	1.5	27.8
Oatmeal, dry	1 cup	>	166.2	5.9	3.5	28.1
Spinach	½ cup	>	4.2	0.5	0.1	0.6
Blueberries	1 cup	>	85.5	1	0.5	21.8
Whey protein isolate	~1 scoop	>	71.9	17.6	0.1	0.1
TOTAL		>	470.3	30.2	5.7	78.4

3   SALMON BURGER

	Serving	Energy (cal)	Protein (g)	Fat (g)	Carbs (g)
Wild sockeye salmon	6 oz	223	38	8	0
Whole-wheat bun	1 each	132	0	1.6	22.2
Olive oil	1 tsp	44.9	0	5	0
Garlic	2 cloves	18.2	0.8	0.1	3.9
Avocado	¼ medium	50.7	0.6	4.6	2.2
Lemon juice	1 Tbsp	3.4	0	0	0.8
TOTAL		472.2	39.4	19.3	29.1

4   OVERNIGHT OATS WITH ALMOND BUTTER AND POMEGRANATE

	Serving	Energy (cal)	Protein (g)	Fat (g)	Carbs (g)
Steel cut oats, uncooked	½ cup	300	10	5	54
Milk, 2% fat	1 cup	127.5	8.5	5	12.3
Banana	1 medium	58.2	0.6	0.2	14.1
Pomegranate	½ medium	49.8	1	0.7	11.2
Maple syrup	1 Tbsp	52	0	0	13.4
Almond butter	1 Tbsp	94.2	3.2	7.8	3.2
TOTAL		681.7	23.3	18.7	108.2

5   SWEET POTATO SMOOTHIE AND A SPORTS DRINK

	Serving	Energy (cal)	Protein (g)	Fat (g)	Carbs (g)
Isotonic sports drink	~25 oz	217.5	0	0	50.3
Sweet potato	1 medium	102.6	2.3	0.2	23.6
Banana	½ medium	58.2	0.6	0.2	14.1
Orange	1 medium	69	1	0.3	17.4
Rice milk	1 cup	90	1	2.5	13
Turmeric powder	1 tsp	17.7	0.4	0.5	3.2
Whey protein isolate	~1 scoop	89.9	22	0.2	0.1
Chia seeds	1 Tbsp	72.9	2.5	4.6	6.3
TOTAL		717.8	29.8	8.5	128

6 BARLEY "RISOTTO" WITH TURKEY, BEANS, AND ZUCCHINI

	Serving		Energy (cal)	Protein (g)	Fat (g)	Carbs (g)
Olive oil	2 tsp	>	89.7	0	10	0
Pearled barley, cooked	1½ cups	>	290	5.3	1	66.5
Skinless turkey breast	3 oz	>	125	25.6	1.8	0
Green beans	1 cup	>	43.8	2.3	0.35	9.9
Zucchini, sliced	2 cups	>	31.5	4.1	0.6	4.7
Chives	1 tsp	>	1.7	0.2	0	0.2
Soy sauce	1 Tbsp	>	6.5	0.5	0	1.2
Semi-dry white wine	1 oz	>	6	0	0	1.5
TOTAL		>	594.2	38	13.75	84

SOCCER DAILY TOTAL

Meal		Energy (cal)	Protein (g)	Fat (g)	Carbs (g)
1	>	489	14.3	14.7	89.8
2	>	470.3	30.2	5.7	78.4
3	>	472.2	39.4	19.3	29.1
4	>	681.7	23.3	18.7	108.2
5	>	717.8	29.8	8.5	128
6	>	594.2	38	13.75	84
TOTAL	>	3,425.20	185.6	92.95	517.5

To replenish carbohydrates, which provide almost 70 percent of the energy needed in soccer, this diet makes use of sweet potatoes. These tubers are also a rich source of protein, fats, and fat-soluble vitamins. A sweet potato's potassium helps maintain the balance of fluid and electrolytes in the body. And the iron and calcium it provides help proper blood circulation and bone density. Thanks to its fiber, complex carbohydrates, protein, fat, vitamins A, B, C, E, and K, and other macro- and micronutrients, the sweet potato ranks near the top of the list of nutritious vegetables. What's more, a sweet potato can also be used during a weight-loss diet because it quickly gives a feeling of satiety, reducing the risk of overeating.

Sweet potatoes contain about 50 percent more nutrients than other potatoes such as Yukons or russets. And despite the name, sweet potatoes can be used in the pre-workout period because they have a moderate glycemic index. They therefore help stabilize blood-sugar levels. Finally, sweet potatoes also play a role in the reduction of insulin resistance.

A soccer player's diet should also include fish. Besides the wholesome proteins that fish provides, it offers healthy fatty acids—mainly omega-3s, which the body is unable to produce. Salmon is a great example of such a fish. Its omega-3 and omega-6 fatty acids are invaluable to our health. They protect against heart disease and relieve joint pain. Just 100 grams (3.5 ounces) of salmon is enough to provide a healthy dose of omega-3 and a similar amount of omega-6, which prevents infections and accelerates wound healing. In addition to valuable fatty acids, salmon contains B vitamins, which are responsible for the proper functioning of the nervous system, vision, and the heart.

It is best to buy wild Alaskan salmon because these products are the cleanest options. Smoked salmon is acceptable but should not be eaten in large quantities because it contains carcinogenic nitrosamines that arise when it is smoked.

Before training, eat a meal that will not overload your digestive system and at the same time will provide the necessary energy. The overnight oats with banana and pomegranate offers an adequate supply of carbohydrates. To slow down absorption of carbs, add healthy fats in the form of almond butter.

A pre-workout meal can benefit from a small amount of fat, but fat should be avoided in a meal immediately after training, as glycogen resynthesis would slow down.

Long-Distance Running

Endurance efforts such as long-distance running are fueled primarily by the aerobic energy system (the main source of energy is body fat) and usually do not cause buildup of lactate, or "lactic acid" as it's often referred to—particularly in highly trained athletes. But running will require moments of higher intensity, such as on hills, during a trail run, or when pushing the pace during a race. In these efforts, a well-trained runner could develop high concentrations of lactate—perhaps more than a less fit individual. The difference, though, is that the well-trained athlete can better manage or clear the lactate. Proper fueling will enable runners of all abilities to perform at their optimal level and improve their ability to run at higher paces.

Depending on the distances run and the frequency of training, the amount of carbohydrates in the runner's diet can range from 4 to 10 grams per kilogram of body weight per day (about 1.8–4.5 g/lb). The lower value will apply to a person training leisurely two to three times per week, while 10 grams of carbohydrates is appropriate for a dozen or so hours of training each week.

The proportion of protein also depends on the frequency of workouts because the more often you train, the faster you need to regenerate your muscles, and therefore a larger proportion of amino acids is necessary. The complete range of recommended protein intake spans from 1.2 to 2 grams per kilogram of body weight per day (0.55–0.90 g/lb). Usually, 1.6–1.9 grams per kilogram are sufficient for most runners, with the exception of marathoners and ultrarunners, for whom the protein share in the preparation period may slightly exceed 2 grams per kilogram. Fats are also important to the diet, especially because during long runs they are the primary source of energy. Fats also build cell membranes, so without adequate amounts of healthy fats in the diet, regeneration of the body will be stunted.

Long-Distance Running

The following sample meal plan was designed for a female 150-pound runner at 32 years of age; she trains for a marathon in the evenings.

1 BANANA PANCAKES WITH JAM AND COTTAGE CHEESE

	Serving	Energy (cal)	Protein (g)	Fat (g)	Carbs (g)
Strawberry jam, reduced sugar	¼ cup	103	0	0	25.6
Cottage cheese, 2% fat	½ cup	91.5	11.8	2.6	5.4
Banana	1 medium	116.4	1.2	0.4	28.2
Whole-wheat flour	½ cup	204	7.9	1.5	43.2
Milk, 2% fat	5 oz.	76.5	5.1	3	7.4
Egg	1 large	70	6.3	4.9	0.3
Coconut oil	1 tsp	43.1	0	5	0
TOTAL		704.5	32.3	17.4	110.1

2 SALAD WITH ROASTED SWEET POTATO, CHICKPEAS, AND TAHINI DRESSING

	Serving	Energy (cal)	Protein (g)	Fat (g)	Carbs (g)
Sweet potato	1 medium	103	2.3	0.2	23.6
Chickpeas, canned	½ cup	105	5.9	2.3	16.2
Arugula	½ cup	2.5	0.3	0.1	0.4
Pomegranate seeds	¼ cup	58.5	1.2	0.8	13.2
Chili powder	2 tsp	28.2	1.4	1.4	5
Tahini	1 tsp	30.4	0.9	2.8	0.9
TOTAL		327.6	12	7.6	59.3

3   RICE CAKES WITH ALMOND BUTTER AND WATERMELON

	Serving	Energy (cal)	Protein (g)	Fat (g)	Carbs (g)
Multigrain rice cakes	2 each	154.8	3.4	1.4	32
Almond butter	2 Tbsp	122.8	4.2	11.1	3.8
Watermelon, cubed	1 cup	108	1.8	0.3	25.2
TOTAL		385.6	9.4	12.8	61

4   CHILI CON CARNE

	Serving	Energy (cal)	Protein (g)	Fat (g)	Carbs (g)
Chopped tomatoes, canned	1 cup	46	2.4	1	6
Onion	½ small	16.5	0.7	0.2	3.5
Canola oil	1 tsp	45	0	5	0
Corn, canned	½ cup	61	2	1	11.3
Red beans, canned	½ cup	103.2	9.1	0.6	15.5
Beef sirloin, grilled	3 oz.	134.4	24.1	4.2	0
Wild rice, cooked	½ cup (dry)	323	9.6	1	69.4
TOTAL		729.1	47.9	13	105.7

5   PIÑA COLADA SMOOTHIE

	Serving	Energy (cal)	Protein (g)	Fat (g)	Carbs (g)
Kiwi	1 medium	42	0.8	0.4	10.2
Pineapple, chopped	½ cup	82.5	0.9	0.4	21.7
Banana	1 medium	116.4	1.2	0.4	28.2
Coconut milk	2 oz	121.8	1.3	10.8	4.9
Soy milk	8 oz	80	8.5	4.8	0.5
TOTAL		442.7	12.7	16.8	65.5

6   MILLET WITH KALE AND FRIED EGGS

	Serving	Energy (cal)	Protein (g)	Fat (g)	Carbs (g)
Sports drink	~25 oz	217.5	0	0	50.3
Green onion	2 stalks	6.4	0.4	0	1.5
Garlic	1 clove	9.1	0.4	0	2
Eggs	2 large	140	12.5	9.7	0.6
Millet, cooked	1 cup	207	6.1	1.7	41.2
Kale	1 cup	7.2	0.7	0.1	1.2
TOTAL		587.2	20.1	11.5	96.8

LONG-DISTANCE RUNNING DAILY TOTAL

Meal	Energy (cal)	Protein (g)	Fat (g)	Carbs (g)
1	704.5	32.3	17.4	110.1
2	327.6	12	7.6	59.3
3	385.6	9.4	12.8	61
4	729.1	47.9	13	105.7
5	442.7	12.7	16.8	65.5
6	587.2	20.1	11.5	96.8
TOTAL	3,176.70	134.4	79.1	498.4

When planning a diet, your own food preferences are a critical part of the equation: If you like the foods you eat, you're more likely to reach for them and stick to your nutrition plan. Try some new foods to expand your palate while ensuring you're getting the best nutrition. For breakfast, instead of a traditional oatmeal, try the banana pancakes; they're especially great for people who prefer something sweet in the morning. Rice crackers with almond butter, smoothies, and carbohydrate bars will work well as snacks during the day or before training. The best bars are those you make yourself; include various types of whole grains, grain flakes, and dried fruit, with the addition of nuts and seeds. Homemade energy bars are fresher, contain exactly the ingredients you like, and are devoid of artificial sugars, preservatives, and other unhealthy ingredients.

When workouts end in the late evening and even at night, some athletes tend to skip nutritious meals and perhaps only drink water and have a light snack and then go to bed. But that's not the most advisable post-workout habit. After a workout, you always need to refuel and recover, so a post-workout meal, if properly composed, will not translate into an increase in body fat or poor quality of sleep, and it will support the body's regeneration and capacity to train again the following day. Post-workout meals should offer both carbohydrates and protein. Antioxidants are also important, as the reactive forms of oxygen that accumulated during the stress of exercise have a detrimental effect on the muscles.

This sample meal plan includes millet as a source of carbohydrates and B-group vitamins, which improve the functioning of the nervous system. Additionally, millet has alkalizing properties, making it easier to maintain the acid-base balance. It also has iron, but at a low bioavailability not exceeding 10 percent. Millet contains a rather large amount of the amino acid tryptophan, which affects the level of serotonin and thus improves mood. Millet is gluten-free and contains relatively little fiber compared to other whole grains, so it can be used in diets for gluten intolerance or people who have other digestion sensitivities.

Ketogenic Diet

The ketogenic diet shifts the body's use of carbohydrates as the primary energy source to fats, even in daily activity (see Chapter 4, "Fats"). New research has shown that such a diet may be beneficial in weight loss and will not cause loss of strength and power, which is especially important for athletes. Some researchers have found that male cyclists on the ketogenic diet lost weight and experienced improvements in body composition and cholesterol and tri-glyceride levels. Other studies conducted among endurance athletes demonstrated that as a result of using a ketogenic diet for a longer time (more than 20 months) the body further adapts to high fat intake.

How the body responds to low-carb diets is quite complex: Ultrarunners on a ketogenic diet for almost two years had a similar glycogen content when compared to group of athletes with a mixed diet. This is due to the increased production of glucose in the liver during gluconeogenesis, a step in ketone-driven energy production. As the body adapts to the ketogenic diet, it allows the body to save muscle and liver glycogen during exercise, especially if medium-chain fatty acids are present and leaned on more readily for energy production.

High-fat diets may work well among people struggling with autoimmune diseases, insulin resistance, and irritable-bowel syndrome, although research in this area is not conclusive and is still ongoing.

Early in the process of incorporating a ketogenic diet, be prepared for mood variability, drowsiness, loss of strength, lower training results, or irritability. In the first 10 to 14 days, the body runs on the vapors of carbohydrate reserves before it begins to draw energy from ketone bodies.

The ketogenic diet, despite its proven effectiveness for both athletes and anyone trying to lose weight, also has its drawbacks and should not be undertaken without careful planning and perhaps a consultation with your sports dietitian. With the near absence of carbohydrates comes a significant reduction of fiber; selenium levels fall, too, which can weaken the immune system. Severe deficiencies of this element may be manifested by the weakening of the myocardium—the muscular tissue of the heart. Supplements should help maintain adequate levels of both fiber and selenium. Another essential nutrient is carnitine, which is necessary for the energy transformation of fats. It is worth checking its concentration every two months; if carnitine levels drop below your physician's recommendation, then carnitine supplements should be introduced. A ketogenic diet can also substantially reduce other vitamins and minerals, including vitamins C and D, calcium, and magnesium. Monitor your intake and find other ways of acquiring an adequate supply of these important nutrients.

Athletes considering a ketogenic diet should factor in their physical activity. In interval training, HIIT, martial arts, or similar sports, the ketogenic diet may contribute to faster fatigue and less-effective training or longer recovery. Therefore, it is worth considering its application carefully because it is not for everyone. Recall that anaerobic systems must draw on carbohydrates, not fats, so the use of a ketogenic diet in exercise with a lot of anaerobic efforts may not offer the best results.

The ketogenic diet can be used periodically, with interruptions for supplementing the glycogen reserve. As a general rule, follow a ketogenic diet for six to eight weeks, and then for two or three days, introduce a small amount of carbohydrates (in the range of 80–160 grams, depending on body weight). But the success of this diet depends on your well-being and how your body adapts to using ketone bodies as the primary source of energy.

The following sample plan fits the requirements of the ketogenic diet, but remember that everyone may need a different proportion of macronutrients to achieve ketosis. You can check the level of ketone bodies on a regular basis via the urine, but a more effective method will be a blood test.

Ketogenic Diet

Following is a sample ketogenic diet for a 136-pound female runner seeking to reduce fat in the abdomen and thighs and regulate her blood-sugar levels.

1   VEGETABLE OMELETTE

	Serving	Energy (cal)	Protein (g)	Fat (g)	Carbs (g)
Eggs	3 large	210	18.8	14.6	0.9
Coconut oil	2 tsp	86.2	0	9	0
Butter	1 Tbsp	101.8	0.1	11.5	0
Bell pepper, chopped	½ cup	14.9	0.6	0.1	3.5
Onion, chopped	¼ cup	32	0.5	0.1	3.5
Mushrooms, sliced	½ cup	7.7	0.5	0.1	1.1
TOTAL		452.6	20.5	35.4	9

2   AVOCADO, BACON, AND EGG SALAD

	Serving	Energy (cal)	Protein (g)	Fat (g)	Carbs (g)
Avocado	¾ medium	169	2	15.3	7.4
Bacon	2 slices	70	4	6	0
Egg, hard-boiled	1 large	77	6.3	5.3	0.5
Parmesan cheese	1 Tbsp	21	1.4	1.4	0
Romaine lettuce, chopped	1 cup	10	0.7	0	2
Bell pepper, chopped	½ cup	14.9	0.7	0.1	3.5
Pumpkin seeds	1 Tbsp	45	2.47	4	0.9
TOTAL		406.9	17.57	32.1	14.3

3   ZUCCHINI "SPAGHETTI" WITH RIB EYE

	Serving	Energy (cal)	Protein (g)	Fat (g)	Carbs (g)
Zucchini, sliced	2 cups	38.4	2.7	0.7	7
Rib eye, grilled	3 oz	248	22	17	0
White mushrooms, sliced	1 cup	15.4	2.2	0.2	2.3
Garlic	4 cloves	18.2	0.8	0.1	3.9
Butter	2 Tbsp	203.6	0.2	23	0
Canola oil	1 Tbsp	90	0	10	0
TOTAL		613.6	27.9	51	13.2

4   BROCCOLI SALAD

	Serving	Energy (cal)	Protein (g)	Fat (g)	Carbs (g)
Sunflower seeds	3 Tbsp	175.2	6.2	15.5	6
Broccoli florets	2 cups	46.5	4.5	0.6	7.8
Cherry tomatoes	12 medium	22.5	1.4	0.3	5.4
TOTAL		244.2	12.1	16.4	19.2

5   COCONUT FLOUR PANCAKES

	Serving	Energy (cal)	Protein (g)	Fat (g)	Carbs (g)
Egg	1 large	70	6.3	4.9	0.3
Baking powder	½ tsp	1	0	0	0
Coconut oil	1 Tbsp	129.3	0	15	0
Cream, half & half	¼ cup	73.8	1.9	6.2	2.8
Coconut flour	¼ cup	123.9	4.9	3.6	16.5
Ground flaxseed	1 Tbsp	30.1	3.7	1.7	3.5
TOTAL		428.1	16.8	31.4	23.1

KETOGENIC DAILY TOTAL				
Meal	Energy (cal)	Protein (g)	Fat (g)	Carbs (g)
1 >	452.6	20.5	35.4	9
2 >	406.9	17.57	32.1	14.3
3 >	613.6	27.9	51	13.2
4 >	244.2	12.1	16.4	19.2
5 >	428.1	16.8	31.4	23.1
TOTAL >	2,145.40	94.87	166.3	78.8

Cheat Meal

Even with the greatest intentions, we sometimes stray from our nutritional goals and allow ourselves a food that isn't quite up to our usual standards. Call it a cheat meal. Athletes might find themselves eating pizza, ice cream, desserts, chips, or other foods that in fact have no place in an active person's daily diet. Giving ourselves an occasional "food break" can be an acceptable practice—especially for the sake of your mental well-being. Of course, that's nearly all these foods are good for, but that's okay once in a while.

Be careful that the cheat meal doesn't grow into an entire cheat day, though. It will wreak havoc on you because if the body receives large amounts of simple sugars, solid fats, empty calories, and too much alcohol, nothing good can result from this; nothing you've eaten in a cheat day will support all the important functions athletes needs to keep their body running well. A cheat day may upset the body's metabolism for the next two to three days, even though you are already eating healthily again. And junk food is known to bring on abdominal pain, diarrhea, constipation, digestive problems, and sometimes headaches; all of these side effects will make it difficult to exercise the next day.

If an athlete must eat cheat meals, he or she should limit them to two per week. Of course, the unhealthy meal should be counted toward the daily calorie and nutrient count and not be an additional supply of calories that day.

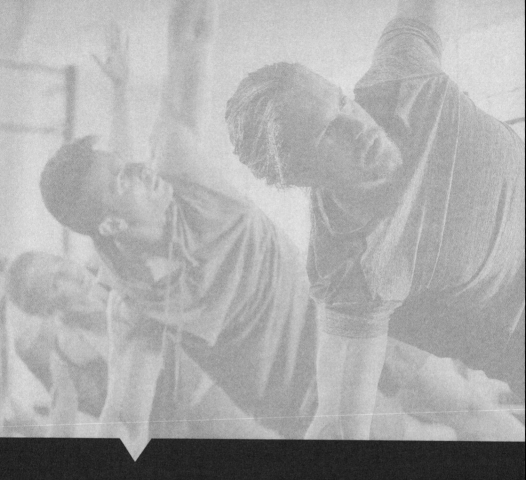

7 | RECIPES

Coconut Pancakes with Mango Mousse

Here's a healthy snack for athletes new to cooking. These pancakes are ideally suited for workday lunches, breakfasts, or pre-workout meals (but give yourself adequate digestion time). This recipe makes more than one serving.

3 eggs

¼ cup coconut flour

1 teaspoon stevia (or other low-calorie sweetener)

5 ounces plus 2½ tablespoons coconut milk

1 tablespoon coconut oil

½ mango

1 teaspoon cinnamon

---

1. Whisk eggs with the flour, sweetener, and 5 ounces coconut milk. The batter should be slightly thicker than for ordinary pancakes. **2.** Pour ¼ cup batter into a hot pan coated with some of the coconut oil (reserve some oil for cooking the remaining pancakes). **3.** Prepare the mousse: Blend mango with 2½ tablespoons coconut milk and cinnamon. Spread mousse on the cooked pancakes.

PROTEIN 29 g • **FAT** 69 g • **CARBS** 50 g • **CAL** 900

All recipes make one serving unless otherwise noted.

Fruit and Oatmeal Crumble

This is a nice alternative to ordinary oatmeal. You can use various seasonal fruits that are good sources of antioxidants.

½ cup rolled oats

1 tablespoon maple syrup

2 teaspoons coconut oil

1 cup raspberries

1 cup strawberries, halved

2 small nectarines, chopped

½ cup Greek yogurt

---

1. Coarsely chop rolled oats in a blender. Mix in syrup and coconut oil. **2.** Spread fruit in a medium baking dish and sprinkle with oat mixture. **3.** Bake in a preheated oven at 325°F for 20 minutes, until golden. Serve with Greek yogurt.

PROTEIN 17 g • **FAT** 17 g • **CARBS** 73 g • **CAL** 490

Rice and Millet Pancakes

Pancakes are a good option for those who prefer sweet breakfasts, and this recipe offers a more nutritious version than plain white-flour pancakes. You can use up leftover rice or millet from another recipe. A breakfast with these pancakes will be tasty and healthy—great for an athlete.

⅓ cup cooked white rice

½ cup cooked millet

2 eggs

3 tablespoons amaranth flour

2 tablespoons corn flour

½ cup 2% milk

3 teaspoons clarified butter, melted (divided)

---

1. Bring cooked grains to room temperature. **2.** Mix all ingredients. **3.** Cook pancakes on a flat pan or griddle with 1 teaspoon butter.

PROTEIN 2 g • **FAT** 25 g • **CARBS** 79 g • **CAL** 660

Millet Pudding with Peanut Butter and Pomegranate

An alternative to plain oatmeal, this is a tasty, colorful, and energizing breakfast.

¼ cup millet, dry
¾ cup 2% milk, divided
1 tablespoon peanut butter
1 small banana
Seeds from ¼ fresh pomegranate
1 teaspoon maple syrup

1. Put millet in a strainer and rinse thoroughly with hot tap water. **2.** Pour millet into a saucepan with about half of the milk, cover, and bring to a boil. **3.** Reduce to low heat and cook for about 15 minutes, until the grains absorb all the liquid. **4.** Add the remaining milk and peanut butter, mix, and heat a little longer. **5.** Transfer to a blender, add banana and blend to a smooth mousse. **6.** Pour into a bowl and sprinkle with pomegranate seeds. **7.** Top with maple syrup.

PROTEIN 17 g • **FAT** 16 g • **CARBS** 89 g • **CAL** 545

Chocolate-Date Butter

This spread is perfect for sandwiches, but it's also tasty with pancakes or smoothies before a workout. This recipe makes more than one serving.

- ½ cup cashews
- ½ cup canned coconut milk
- 1 teaspoon cocoa powder
- 4 Medjool dates

1. Grind nuts into a powder. **2.** Combine nut powder with milk, cocoa powder, and dates (if dried, soak them ahead of time to rehydrate them) in blender and puree until creamy. **3.** Store in a cool place for a maximum of 5–6 days.

PROTEIN 15 g • **FAT** 56 g • **CARBS** 89 g • **CAL** 840

Chocolate Smoothie with Prunes

This smoothie can be a nice light breakfast or a snack when recovering from a workout.

3 prunes

¼ cup millet

1 cup unsweetened coconut milk

1 tablespoon cocoa powder

1 tablespoon almond butter

1. Fill a container so that water just covers the prunes and soak overnight. **2.** Cook millet according to package directions (or see instructions in Millet Pudding with Peanut Butter and Pomegranate recipe, p. 161). **3.** Add millet to prune/water container (do not drain prunes). **4.** Add remaining ingredients and puree in blender until smooth.

PROTEIN 11 g • **FAT** 16 g • **CARBS** 63 g • **CAL** 412

Quinoa, Banana, and Raspberry Smoothie

This is a fast and energizing snack for those who start their training very early. It also works well for people with sensitivity to gluten.

¼ cup quinoa, dry
1 medium banana
1 cup raspberries
½ cup yogurt
1 cup unsweetened coconut milk

1. Cook quinoa according to package directions. **2.** Combine cooked quinoa with remaining ingredients and puree in blender until smooth. If the smoothie is too thick, add water.

PROTEIN 15 g • FAT 9 g • CARBS 82 g • CAL 430

Strawberry, Rhubarb, and Amaranth Smoothie

Another good option for breakfast, this smoothie is best when strawberries and rhubarb are in season. It works well before training and for people with lactose intolerance.

1 cup diced rhubarb

1 cup strawberries

1 cup unsweetened soy milk

2 tablespoons amaranth flakes

¼ avocado

1. Place diced rhubarb in a pot of water and bring to boil; reduce heat to a simmer, cover, and let cook for 15 minutes. **2.** Strain, reserving some of the water, and let rhubarb cool. **3.** Combine with the remaining ingredients and puree in blender until smooth. Add reserved water as needed to adjust thickness.

PROTEIN 11 g • **FAT** 15 g • **CARBS** 39 g • **CAL** 320

Toast with Beets and Cottage Cheese

A twist on the usual sandwich—this time with healthy beets and cheese. This is a good option for breakfast, but also a light dinner.

1 large or 2 small beets

2 slices whole-grain rye bread

1 clove garlic

2 tablespoons hazelnuts

½ cup low-fat cottage cheese

Salt and pepper

1. Preheat the oven to 350°F. **2.** Wash beets, wrap in aluminum foil, and place on a small pan in the oven. **3.** Bake until tender (check by pricking with a fork; 35–60 minutes). **4.** Toast bread in a sauté pan or in the oven. **5.** Rub toasted bread with a garlic clove cut lengthwise. **6.** Roast hazelnuts in a dry pan for about 5 minutes; when cool, chop coarsely. **7.** Peel beets and cut into thin, long strips using a vegetable peeler. **8.** Arrange beet strips on toasted bread and top with cottage cheese and nuts. Season with salt and pepper.

PROTEIN 24 g • **FAT** 14 g • **CARBS** 51 g • **CAL** 416

Salad with Roasted Beets and Prosciutto

This salad makes a satisfying part of lunch or an afternoon snack. It will keep you feeling full thanks to an ample portion of complete proteins and healthy fats. For active people, beets are a good part of the diet because they improve aerobic capacity.

2 small beets

2 handfuls arugula

¼ avocado, sliced

2 ounces prosciutto

1 tablespoon sunflower seeds

1 teaspoon canola oil

1. Peel beets, cut into slices, place on a baking tray, and bake at 350°F until tender, about 25 minutes. Allow to cool. **2.** Arrange arugula on a plate. **3.** Add beets, avocado, and ham; sprinkle sunflower seeds on top and drizzle with oil.

PROTEIN 22 g ● **FAT** 21 g ● **CARBS** 19 g ● **CAL** 340

Quinoa Salad with Salmon and Grapefruit

The dish is suitable for either lunch or dinner; the grapefruit, although it is a fruit, can be consumed later in the day because it has a low GI. This particular citrus fruit supports the reduction of fat tissue.

1 large grapefruit

¾ cup cooked quinoa

1 cup chopped lettuce

2 teaspoons finely grated grapefruit zest

1 tablespoon olive oil

1 teaspoon honey

Salt and pepper

4 ounces smoked salmon, cut in bite-size pieces

2 tablespoons chopped pecans

---

1. Halve and gently squeeze grapefruit, collecting about a tablespoon of juice; remove grapefruit sections with a knife (retain the membranes). **2.** Place cooked quinoa on a plate and add lettuce and grapefruit sections. **3.** In a small bowl, mix grapefruit juice with zest, olive oil, honey, and salt and pepper to make a vinaigrette. **4.** Add salmon to the salad and pour vinaigrette as desired. Sprinkle with pecans.

PROTEIN 30 g • **FAT** 30 g • **CARBS** 43 g • **CAL** 531

Quinoa with Turkey and Vegetables

This quick dish is tasty either hot or cold. It is well suited as a lunch at work, as well as a meal before an evening workout thanks to its carbohydrates with a medium glycemic index. Quinoa is also a good solution for people eliminating gluten from their diet.

1 cup cooked quinoa

3 ounces turkey breast

1 cup sliced zucchini

4 medium carrots, peeled and sliced

1 tablespoon coconut oil

1 clove garlic, peeled and crushed

Salt

Juice of 1 lemon

½ teaspoon ground turmeric

½ teaspoon dried thyme

---

1. Cut turkey meat into small cubes and cut zucchini into half-slices. **2.** Pour about 1 tablespoon oil into a large heated sauté pan; add crushed garlic. **3.** Add turkey and sprinkle it with salt; fry briefly and then add carrots and zucchini. **4.** Drizzle with lemon juice and add thyme and turmeric. Stir gently and sauté until meat is tender and vegetables are cooked but still crisp. **5.** When turkey and vegetables are ready, add quinoa. Mix everything, sautéing briefly. **6.** Adjust the salt and sprinkle with more thyme before serving if desired.

PROTEIN 30 g • **FAT** 17 g • **CARBS** 75 g • **CAL** 560

Chicken with Lentils and Vegetables

This high-protein dish will work well as a recovery meal or in a weight-loss diet, as it keeps you feeling satiated for a long time.

¼ cup red or green lentils

2 medium carrots

1 small parsnip

3 medium celery stalks

1 leek

1 tablespoon canola oil

3 ounces grilled or roasted chicken breast, diced

Salt and pepper

Chili flakes (optional)

1 teaspoon parsley

---

1. Rinse lentils by adding them to a pot with at least ½ cup of water and bringing to a boil. After about a minute, strain and rinse with cold water. **2.** Return rinsed lentils to the pot, add ¾ cup fresh water, and cook on low heat until tender. (Red lentils cook in about 20 minutes; green lentils will cook in 30 minutes or more.) **3.** Wash, peel, and slice carrots and parsnips; slice celery and leek cross-wise. **4.** Heat oil in a large sauté pan and add vegetables. **5.** When nearly tender, add chicken and continue to cook. **6.** Add cooked lentils to the vegetables and chicken mixture and sauté for another minute or two. **7.** Add about 6 ounces of water and stir from time to time. **8.** Add salt and pepper to taste and chili flakes if you like. Sprinkle with parsley.

PROTEIN 34 g • **FAT** 15 g • **CARBS** 73 g • **CAL** 540

Salmon Burgers with Guacamole and Yogurt

Salmon burgers are a healthy alternative to fast-food burgers, and they're almost as fast to prepare. Thanks to the healthy fats in the fish, this burger will keep you feeling full despite its moderate size.

4 ounces fresh salmon

Salt and pepper

1 teaspoon olive oil

2 small whole-grain rolls

¼ ripe avocado

2 teaspoons lemon juice (divided)

2 cloves garlic, minced (divided)

¼ cup nonfat Greek yogurt

2 or 3 lettuce leaves

1. Shred the raw salmon with a food processor, but don't let the fish become too finely ground. **2.** Add salt and pepper to fish, mix, and form two small patties. **3.** Heat oil in frying pan over medium heat until it shimmers. **4.** Place patties on the hot pan. **5.** Once well browned around the edges (4–6 minutes), flip and cook for about the same amount of time and remove from pan. **6.** Grill rolls in pan or warm them in oven. **7.** To prepare guacamole and yogurt spreads, use a fork to smash avocado with 1 teaspoon lemon juice, half of the garlic, and salt and pepper. **8.** In a separate bowl, mix yogurt with the remaining garlic and 1 teaspoon lemon juice. **9.** Prepare the burgers as desired: Each burger can get a little of each spread, or use guacamole for one burger and yogurt for the other. Top each with lettuce.

PROTEIN 40 g • **FAT** 14 g • **CARBS** 43 g • **CAL** 500

Rice Noodles with Miso and Salmon

This noodle dish is easy to prepare and good at home or on the go. It contains a healthy mix of all macronutrients and keeps you feeling satisfied.

½ cup rice noodles

1 teaspoon coconut oil

1 chili pepper, diced

1-inch section fresh ginger root, peeled and grated

1 tablespoon sesame seeds

1 tablespoon miso

1 tablespoon soy sauce

2 tablespoons lime juice, divided

6 ounces salmon, cut into 1-inch cubes

1 teaspoon sesame oil

1 tablespoon minced fresh chives

½ teaspoon minced fresh cilantro

---

1. Cook noodles according to package directions, strain noodles, and chop once or twice. **2.** Heat coconut oil in a sauté pan or wok on low heat. Add chili pepper, grated ginger, and sesame seeds and cook briefly until fragrant. **3.** Add miso paste, soy sauce, and half of the lime juice. **4.** Bring to moderate heat for about a minute, stirring constantly. **5.** Add salmon cubes and fry on each side just until the fish cooks through (about 2 minutes). **6.** Add cooked noodles and sprinkle with sesame oil, chives, and cilantro; add remaining lime to taste.

PROTEIN 41 g • **FAT** 21 g • **CARBS** 72 g • **CAL** 640

Rice Noodles with Beef

Beef is a very good source of iron, which improves an athlete's performance. With its combination of carbohydrates and protein, this dish is an ideal lunch or dinner for the active person.

5 ounces beef sirloin

½ cup rice noodles

4 stalks green onions

1 tablespoon soy sauce

1 tablespoon brown sugar

1-inch section fresh ginger root, peeled and grated

2 cloves garlic, minced

1 tablespoon coconut oil, divided

1 tablespoon dried red pepper flakes

¼ red or green pepper, cut into thin strips

1 chili pepper, cut into thin strips (optional)

5 mint leaves, chopped

Juice from ½ lime

---

1. Cut sirloin across the grain into very thin slices. **2.** Cook noodles according to package directions, drain, and set aside. **3.** Chop green onions, separating the green ends from the white. **4.** Mix soy sauce with brown sugar in a small dish. **5.** Gently cook ginger and garlic in ½ tablespoon coconut oil in a wok or frying pan, about 4 minutes. **6.** Add remaining ½ tablespoon oil, the white pieces of green onions, pepper flakes, and red or green pepper. Stir for about a minute. **7.** Add meat to pan and fry for about 1 minute, until the meat turns to brown. **8.** Add chili pepper, if using, and the cooked rice noodles. **9.** Cook for 1 minute, stirring continuously. **10.** Pour in the soy sauce mixture, remaining green onion, and mint. Mix thoroughly. **11.** Sprinkle with lime juice and serve.

PROTEIN 33 g • **FAT** 20 g • **CARBS** 59 g • **CAL** 540

Scallops with Lentils and Carrots

For the adventurous eater and cook, this dish will inspire. It's the perfect meal for an athlete thanks to its healthy supply of lean protein, beta-carotene, and healthy fats.

½ cup red or green lentils, dry

2 medium carrots

2 tablespoons coconut oil, divided

2 cloves garlic, minced

1-inch section fresh ginger root, peeled and grated

1 tablespoon almond butter

1 tablespoon miso

1 tablespoon soy sauce

2 tablespoons peanuts

4 ounces scallops

---

1. Rinse the lentils, then place in pot with 3 cups water. Bring to a boil. **2.** Cover, reduce heat, and cook 20–40 minutes, until lentils are tender and have absorbed all of the water. **3.** Peel carrots; then continue using the peeler to make thin strips. **4.** Heat a tablespoon of coconut oil in a wok or frying pan, toss in the garlic and ginger, add carrots, almond butter, miso, and soy sauce, and stir-fry gently for about 4 minutes. **5.** Move the carrot mixture to the side of the pan, toss the peanuts into the open side of the pan, and cook until they turn light brown. Move peanuts to the side. **6.** Add a second tablespoon of coconut oil into the empty space and set the scallops in carefully, leaving space between them. **7.** Let scallops cook, untouched, 4–5 minutes; then turn them over and cook for half the time—about 2 minutes. **8.** Combine scallops with carrot mixture and stir-fry for 1 minute. **9.** Add cooked lentils and gently combine all ingredients.

PROTEIN 37 g • **FAT** 25 g • **CARBS** 62 g • **CAL** 600

Cod with Sweet Potato Fries

This dish will work well both before and after a workout. Before a workout, you can use more potatoes, and after, use less fat for a more effective recovery.

2 medium sweet potatoes

Salt and pepper

1 tablespoon fresh rosemary leaves, finely chopped

1 tablespoon canola oil

4 ounces fresh cod fillet

1 teaspoon clarified butter

---

1. Heat oven to 425°F. **2.** Cut sweet potatoes lengthwise into ½-inch thick slices. Stack two or three slices at a time and cut again lengthwise, making fries. **3.** Place sweet potatoes in a bowl; sprinkle with salt and pepper. Add rosemary and oil and toss to distribute seasoning. **4.** Put fries on a baking pan, keeping space between individual fries, and put pan in oven. **5.** Set timer for 20 minutes. Meanwhile, top fish with salt, pepper, and clarified butter. **6.** With 5 minutes remaining on timer, turn on broiler and add fish to the pan. Bake for 5 minutes or until fish is cooked through and tender.

PROTEIN 25 g • **FAT** 19 g • **CARBS** 48 g • **CAL** 468

Shrimp with Zucchini Ribbons and Rice

This tasty main dish is good almost any time of day, but it's not recommended as a post-workout meal. Despite its healthy dose of protein, it contains too many fats that will delay post-workout regeneration.

1 medium zucchini

1 teaspoon canola oil

½ cup onion, chopped

2 cloves garlic, thinly sliced

½-inch section fresh ginger root, peeled and finely grated

1 chili pepper, seeded and cut into strips

1 teaspoon curry powder

5 ounces frozen shrimp, cleaned and shelled

½ cup (canned) coconut milk

¾ cup cooked wild rice

Salt and pepper

Fresh cilantro

1. Wash the zucchini thoroughly but do not peel it. **2.** Shave zucchini into strips with a vegetable peeler and blanch in boiling, lightly salted water (1–2 minutes). **3.** Drain zucchini and place the strips on a paper towel. **4.** Heat oil in a large sauté pan over medium heat. **5.** Add onion, garlic, ginger, chili pepper, and curry powder to pan and sauté for about 1 minute. **6.** Add shrimp; turn up heat and sauté for about 3 minutes. **7.** Pour in coconut milk and bring to a boil. **8.** Add cooked rice to pan and continue cooking shrimp mixture for 5 minutes. **9.** Remove from the heat and add zucchini strips. Season with salt and pepper to taste. Serve sprinkled with fresh cilantro.

PROTEIN 33 g • **FAT** 30 g • **CARBS** 50 g • **CAL** 580

Tuna Steak with Spinach

This main course, rich in omega-3 fatty acids, can also be a pre-workout meal.

1 large sweet potato
4 ounces fresh tuna fillet
Salt and pepper
1 teaspoon finely chopped fresh rosemary leaves
2 teaspoons canola oil, divided
½ cup frozen spinach, thawed, rinsed, and patted dry
2 tablespoons raisins
1 teaspoon olive oil
1 tablespoon pine nuts

---

1. Prepare sweet potato fries as instructed in the Cod with Sweet Potato Fries recipe (p. 175). **2.** Rinse and dry tuna fillet, season with salt, pepper, and rosemary, and coat with a thick layer of oil. **3.** Heat a sauté pan to medium-high heat and add remaining oil. Add fish to pan and let cook for about 1–2 minutes on each side. It is most flavorful when tuna stays pink in the middle—medium or medium rare—but cook to a temperature that you are comfortable with. **4.** Remove tuna from pan and set aside. **5.** Lower heat and add spinach and raisins with 1 teaspoon olive oil for 1–2 minutes, stirring occasionally. Put spinach mixture on a plate, place the tuna on top, and sprinkle with pine nuts. Serve with sweet potato fries.

PROTEIN 36 g • **FAT** 20 g • **CARBS** 57 g • **CAL** 550

Chicken and Vegetable Skewers

Skewers or kebabs are great when cooking for two or more because they're fun to make, and you can prepare them exactly to order. You can grill some whole-grain bread or flatbread to accompany the skewers. These additional carbs will replenish glycogen supplies while the chicken provides muscles with protein.

5 ounces boneless, skinless chicken breast

1 teaspoon canola oil

2 teaspoons curry powder (or other spice as desired)

½ large red pepper, cut into 8 pieces

½ large onion, cut into 8 pieces

4 small mushrooms, cut in half

6 cherry tomatoes

---

1. Cut chicken into 6 to 8 pieces, lightly drizzle with oil, and coat with curry powder. **2.** Smear two or three skewers with canola oil and slide chicken and vegetables on, fitting them tightly. **3.** Grill skewers for about 5 minutes or wrap them in foil and roast in a 350°F oven for 15 minutes.

PROTEIN 36 g • **FAT** 7 g • **CARBS** 16 g • **CAL** 270

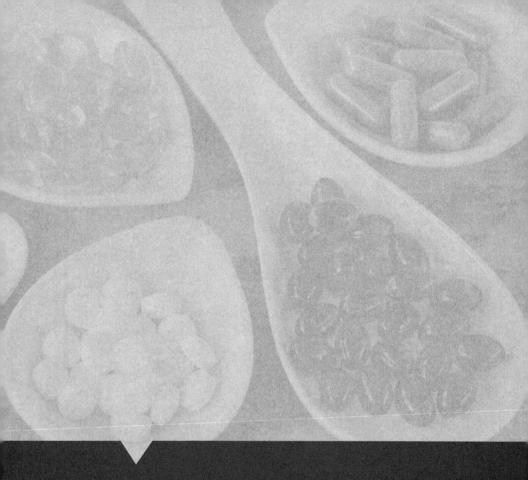

8 NUTRITIONAL SUPPLEMENTS

A properly balanced diet is the most important element of an athlete's nutrition plan. It should provide the body with all the necessary substrates, minerals, and vitamins. However, it can be difficult, and sometimes impossible, for some people to consume all the correct foods within even a 4,000- or 5,000-calorie diet. For this reason, dietary supplements are becoming more and more popular. Many people misuse them, though, forgetting that they are just a supplement to the diet, not a mainstay. Taken with care, supplements can have a beneficial effect on the athlete's body: strength, endurance, speed, and post-workout recovery.

Each year the supplement market grows, with new compounds constantly emerging. Unfortunately, they are often not as effective as they would seem. Although an entire book could be written on supplements, we will discuss only the most important and most popular types, whose effects on the body have been confirmed by numerous scientific studies and the experience of coaches, trainers, and nutritionists.

Branched-Chain Amino Acids

Branched-chain amino acids (BCAAs) are a popular supplement used for their ability to aid regeneration after a workout. They are formed by three amino acids: leucine, isoleucine, and valine, which account for about one-third of all muscle proteins. The human body cannot create these three amino acids by itself (they are essential amino acids), so they need to be supplied from food.

While most amino acids undergo changes in the liver, BCAAs are used directly in the muscles. After a physical effort, the body has an energy deficit, which causes a decrease in leucine levels and a deficiency of branched-chain amino acids. A significant part of leucine is obtained through the degradation of the body's own proteins. BCAA supplements are taken to fill that need instead (in fact, BCAA is currently one of the most popular supplements used by athletes).

Scientific research has confirmed that these amino acids have anabolic and anticatabolic effects and significantly affect the regeneration of the body,

CASE STUDY A Teenager Discovers That Misusing Supplements Does More Harm than Good

Andrew, 14, had designed a diet so that he would gain muscle mass. He had been training in the gym for six months under the guidance of his 18-year-old brother. Andrew was determined to quickly improve his physique, as he was quite frail for his age (he weighed 93 pounds with a height of 4'10"). Despite his youth, he was very well read and knew a lot about diet and supplements. Even after learning that teenagers should approach strength training and nutrition very differently than adults would, he wanted to do anything he could to gain muscle mass. Looking up to his muscular brother, he would not follow the more common advice that someone his age should focus on body weight exercises and general athleticism like playing sports. His family supported his decision, too.

Andrew had a long list of supplements that he planned on taking. It included, among others, creatine, arginine, BCAA, protein supplements, and testosterone booster. He also wanted to eat a high-calorie diet, well over what would be recommended for his age and strength training regimen.

After a year of sticking to his own high-calorie diet, which also included copious amounts of daily supplements, Andrew had gained a lot of weight but had not increased his muscle mass. He had health problems, kidney problems, and abdominal pain. His mother blamed the supplements, and Andrew was finally forced to stop taking them.

THE FIX: Education was crucial for Andrew to modify his diet and supplement use. A properly balanced diet—without supplements—was enough to cover his caloric demand, even with his high level of physical activity. From a physiological point of view, until he would begin to produce the right amount of testosterone, strength training would not bring the results he hoped for. It was simply a matter of his age.

RESULTS: Andrew set aside the supplements and focused on a healthy, balanced diet with a more appropriate caloric intake (substantial but not as high as before). After three months, Andrew saw significant improvement in his health, well-being, and physique. ∎

especially after intense training. In people studied who gave up physical exercise and stayed in bed for six days, protein synthesis decreased. But for those subjects who increased BCAA intake from 25 grams to 50 grams per day, protein synthesis in the muscles stabilized and did not further decline. In studies conducted on athletes in strength sports, it was found that a five-week training program with weights caused a decrease in BCAA levels by 20 percent (despite consumption of 1.26 grams of protein per kilogram of body weight). Subsequent studies confirmed that taking BCAA (in which 35 percent was leucine) before exercise minimized the risk of muscle protein degradation.

In athletes taking BCAA before, during, and after training, their bodies' anabolic response was 3.5 times stronger than in the group taking a placebo. In another study, a group of people who trained for strength and received BCAA before and after training for eight weeks were compared with people training in the same way but taking a placebo. It turned out that in the first group, the increase in body weight was 1,000 grams, and in the control group, 750 grams. Among the people taking BCAA, fat loss was also higher (4.5 kilograms compared to 500 grams in the control group). In addition, an increase in the strength of thigh muscles was observed in 22 percent of the BCAA group compared to 18 percent in the placebo group.

Branched-chain amino acids do not degrade in the gastrointestinal tract and in the liver, so when taken orally, they enter the bloodstream and muscles quickly.

Determining a recommended dose is an individual matter, but it has been shown that an intake of 2 grams of BCAA before and after training slows the catabolic processes of muscle tissue during and after exercise. Other researchers say that BCAA should be taken in the amount of 0.1–0.2 grams for every kilogram of body weight, with the maximum daily dose not exceeding 50 grams.

Glutamine

Glutamine belongs to the group of conditionally essential amino acids—those that are created in the body but not always at levels high enough to fulfill their role. With high training loads, it is reasonable to supplement glutamine so that muscles can regenerate as much as necessary.

Glutamine is the most highly concentrated amino acid in the human body; it constitutes over 60 percent of all free amino acids in the muscles. It is necessary for many physiological functions in the brain, immune system, digestive tract, and muscles. This puts high demands on our glutamine reserves. The brain and the immune system are the first to benefit from this supply, so when the body undergoes heavy physical training, the glutamine resources may be too small to also support the muscles that now need it for recovery. At such times, it is helpful to reach for a glutamine supplement. For active people, glutamine is important mainly as a post-workout regenerator and anticatabolic supplement, but it will also improve conditions in the intestines, which will translate into a better absorption of other nutrients.

The supplement L-glutamine improves the activity of the gastrointestinal tract, increases the production of glycogen in the liver, and is used to convert ammonia to urea. L-glutamine also significantly affects other functions, such as protein synthesis, production of GABA (an important neurotransmitter), cell growth, and biosynthesis of DNA and RNA. L-glutamine stimulates the cells of the immune system and protects cells against foodborne and airborne toxins.

Glutamine is an essential component in the production of the antioxidant and detoxifier, glutathione. Glutathione, in turn, improves the efficiency and endurance of the body, which is why the appropriate amount of glutamine as a component of glutathione is important.

Less than 10 grams of glutamine is found in an average daily diet, and this amount may be too low. Moderate to heavy physical activity adds to the burden on glutamine supplies. During periods of increased training, glutamine is released from skeletal muscles into the bloodstream, and its intracellular concentration decreases by up to 50 percent.

Supplementation can therefore help return glutamine to desirable levels. It is difficult to determine the optimal dose of glutamine, as there are many discrepancies in the research. But current studies support the general recommendation that physically active people can take 15–40 grams of a glutamine supplement. Such amounts are enough to protect the muscle's own glutamine, maintain intestinal integrity, provide energy for cells, improve the nitrogen balance, and thus help maintain the overall biological balance of the body. Intake should not exceed 40 grams per day because some side effects may develop at amounts greater, including a stress on the kidneys.

To raise the level of glutamine in the body, it is best to use small doses, such as 4–5 grams two to three times per day, taken at intervals of 90–120 minutes. Recent research shows that supplementation with L-glutamine in the amount of 0.3 grams per kilogram of body weight accelerates regeneration and reduces muscle soreness after training; with this recommendation, a person weighing 175 pounds would take 24 grams of glutamine. Interestingly, the study showed greater effectiveness of L-glutamine in men than in women.

The most common form of the supplement is synthetically produced L-glutamine. The natural form of glutamine is a peptide derived from plant sources. Also available is N-acetyl-L-glutamine (NAG). There are also glutamine precursors (the initial substances necessary for the production of glutamine), such as glutamic acid (as a neurotransmitter, in excess it may be detrimental to the cells of the nervous system) and glutamine alpha-ketoglutarate (AKG).

NAG is rapidly absorbed, and it is not converted into inactive metabolites when it reaches the muscle cell, so it immediately increases the concentration of active glutamine, which directly affects muscle regeneration. It is much more stable and more durable than other forms of glutamine. Glutamine AKG is one of the most advanced glutamine precursors; it is very useful in the rapid transport of nutrients to muscle cells.

Arginine

The amino acid arginine is very important for athletes, who need more of it than nonathletes. Although the body can produce it, some supplementation is helpful. Arginine is involved in the synthesis of creatine, nitric oxide, ornithine, citrulline, and glutamate—substances that are also important for an athlete. Arginine acts as an antioxidant and improves the functioning of the immune system, thus reducing the risk of injury and illness. In addition, as a basic amino acid, it participates in the regulation of blood pH levels. Arginine is found in proteins of animal and vegetable origin, and its daily supply from these sources ranges from 3 grams to 6 grams. Absorption of arginine takes place in the small intestine; about 40 percent of absorbed arginine is degraded and excreted from the body.

Arginine is a precursor to the production of nitric oxide, which is important for an athlete as it dilates blood vessels. In turn, more nutrients, hormones, and oxygen can be delivered to the muscles in a shorter amount of time. It is also an effective regenerator of damaged muscle fibers and an important factor in healing wounds and inflammations, which are not uncommon in competitive sports.

As a precursor to creatine, arginine's presence contributes to muscle strength and better regeneration after training. And when creatine is abundant, it supports the availability of phosphocreatine, which leads to faster ATP resynthesis. And with more ATP available, the athlete will have more power and strength.

Arginine does have some drawbacks, though. With the increased blood flow, there is a chance that some muscles can experience swelling (for example, in the legs of runners, cyclists, or martial artists), which makes exercise difficult. But other athletes praise this effect, professing that it helps them. If you take arginine supplements, be sure to test it out during regular training periods rather than just before an important competition.

The effectiveness of arginine was demonstrated during the supplementation of 12 grams per day with L-arginine alpha-ketoglutarate (AAKG) for eight weeks. In the group using AAKG, compared to the placebo group, a significant increase in maximum muscle power was observed as well as an increase in arginine concentration in the plasma. The body composition of the subjects in both groups did not change. Note that the optimal dose of arginine may be slightly lower than the amount used in this research.

Other studies found that 9 grams per day is effective without causing any side effects. It was also found that doses of 21 grams and 30 grams per day may cause adverse changes in blood chemistry. Other researchers have shown that oral administration of less than 10 grams of arginine does not always cause an increase in blood flow throughout the muscles. The optimal dose of arginine supplementation will depend on your own body, so test carefully within safe ranges.

Creatine

Creatine is one of the most popular permitted supplements in the world, used by both professional and amateur athletes, most often where strength and increased muscle mass are a priority. This compound has been known since at least 1926, when biochemist Alfred Chanutin stated that oral administration of 10 grams of creatine daily for seven days satisfies its supply in skeletal muscles. Today, there are several varieties of creatine on the market: from monohydrate, malate, citrate, and Kre-Alkalyn to creatine stacks.

Creatine occurs naturally in the body and is composed of three amino acids: methionine, arginine, and glycine. It appears mainly in muscles but also in the brain, heart, and testes. Muscles store 66 percent of their creatine in the form of phosphocreatine and 33 percent as free creatine. It is estimated that, on average, about 120 grams of creatine is stored in human muscles, and with proper training and diet, this amount can be increased to 160 grams.

Creatine, which is the energy carrier in muscle cells, is especially useful in speed-strength disciplines, such as 100-meter sprints, weight lifting, long jump, and the like—any sport where power and speed dominate. In these efforts, the body derives energy from ATP and resynthesizes it quickly, a process in which phosphocreatine is necessary. One nuance of creatine's impact on sprinting, though, is that it doesn't improve sprint efficiency in long-term efforts—for example, finishing kicks in long-distance runs.

It has also been shown that a high concentration of creatine in the muscles stimulates protein synthesis, acting as an anticatabolic and anabolic compound, which encourages faster muscle growth, performance, and regeneration.

The use of creatine monohydrate causes an increase in creatine and phosphocreatine concentrations by up to 40 percent. However, the body's response to creatine can vary, so some people can accumulate more of it than others. In those who have a lower initial creatine concentration (caused by, for example, a vegetarian diet or lower activity of creatine-synthesis enzymes), greater increases in its concentration in the muscles have been observed.

In one study, untrained participants took 24 grams of creatine daily in the first week and then 6 grams (or a placebo) for 15 weeks, and they performed strength exercise routines throughout the study period. After four weeks, all subjects demonstrated an increase in the number of satellite cells (responsible for regeneration) by about 110 percent. The placebo group had a rapid increase in muscle mass for the first four weeks, when they did take creatine, but then their levels plateaued; strength training alone did not affect satellite cell growth.

Recommendations for adequate doses are not standardized. Age, sex, type of sport, and muscle fiber composition all factor into the decision. Type II muscle fibers, the "speed and strength" fibers, absorb more creatine than type I "endurance" fibers. In general, 3–5 grams of creatine supplement per day during general training and up to 20 grams per day during the peak phase (a five to seven day increase of creatine intake to saturate muscles). The International Olympic Committee has not placed creatine on the list of prohibited substances, so it is allowed in sports at any level.

Protein Supplements

Protein supplements are most often used by those who are developing strength and muscle mass. Sometimes we want protein supplies to be topped up as soon as possible, and at other times we want supplies to be released more slowly, so protein supplements with different absorption times have been produced.

Protein-based supplements generally come from one or more of the following sources: milk (whey and casein), soy, or eggs. Whey and casein supplements are the most common. Numerous studies have reported that protein supplements stimulate the synthesis of skeletal muscle proteins, inhibit the breakdown of muscle proteins, and affect the increase of muscles' resistance to exercise. Some researchers found that a dose of 25 grams of protein is sufficient during or immediately after exercise to optimize muscle protein synthesis. They also noted that whey proteins tend to have the greatest efficiency.

Whey

Obtained from milk in two ways (microfiltration or ion exchange), whey has a higher biological value than milk. It's best taken immediately after training because it is quickly digested and easily absorbed. Due to the high concentration of branched-chain amino acids (around 25 percent), it supports regeneration after training and fights catabolic processes (those that degrade biological materials, even muscle tissue). Recent research has shown that whey can be successfully used not only in strength training but also in endurance sports like running and cycling. Three components, or fractions, can be found in whey: whey protein isolate (WPI), whey protein hydrolysate (WPH; hydrolyzed whey protein), and whey protein concentrate. The first two fractions are characterized by a very high bioavailability; whey protein concentrate requires the most time for absorption and contains some carbohydrates.

Hydrolyzed whey protein is a specific type of protein that has already been digested during production. It will work best after training because it is perfect for regeneration and muscle repair. In addition, it has the ability to stimulate the production of insulin, which as an anabolic hormone, affects the growth of muscle mass after training. Hydrolyzed whey does not contain carbohydrates. The isolate, just like the hydrolysate, is a very pure form of protein supplement (over 90 percent pure protein), but its molecules are slightly larger than the hydrolysate form. The isolate causes a sharp increase in amino acids in the blood plasma, which favors the rapid reconstruction of muscle structure, so just like the hydrolysate, it can be used immediately after training. The concentrate, on the other hand, contains proteins with different absorption times. It consists of up to 85 percent pure protein and carbohydrates. This type of protein is popular because it can be used after training (it will be released into the bloodstream more slowly than WPH and WPI), to supplement meals with protein, and also at night, in combination with healthy fats, to limit catabolism.

Researchers compared the effects of ordinary whey protein, hydrolysate, and a placebo on the degree of muscle recovery after eccentric resistance training (muscle-lengthening movements like bicep and hamstring curls). It turned out that in comparison with the placebo and a nonhydrolyzed isolate, the adoption of a single dose (25 grams) of whey protein hydrolysate causes faster regeneration of muscle strength after completing eccentric exercises. The research also confirmed that the protein can accelerate muscle recovery after intense weight training. Moreover, the hydrolysate has a positive effect on increasing muscle performance and endurance.

The effects are even greater when the isolate is used in combination with creatine. This has a significant impact on the development of strength and muscle mass, even in middle-aged and elderly people (48–72 years of age). Other studies have shown that in young men training every day for 12 weeks, consumption of 25 grams of whey protein after training contributed to strengthening stem cells by 35 percent compared to a placebo group, which translated into better muscle recovery.

Hydrolysate is very effective but also the most expensive protein fraction. Its effect on regeneration after training is comparable to that of an isolate, so for athletes on a budget, the use of whey protein isolate will also bring equally good benefits. Hydrolysate can be used by people with lactose intolerance. If you don't want to spend money on several types of protein for different occasions, consider a concentrate that will work at different times of the day (before and after training and overnight).

Casein

Casein, like whey proteins, comes from milk, but its molecules are larger than those in isolate or hydrolysate fractions, so casein takes more time to be digested and absorbed. Casein contains about 20 percent glutamine, which can have a positive effect on muscle regeneration. For this reason, this type of supplement is best used overnight to protect the body from nocturnal catabolism. In comparison with the isolate, it has less influence on anabolic processes, but it definitely limits the rate of protein breakdown (by 34 percent). So casein exhibits primarily protective, anticatabolic properties, but it also positively affects muscular stem cells.

In one experiment, in which for 10 weeks one group of participants taking up a strength training program were administered the protein isolate, and another group took casein, it turned out that the whey protein isolate group had a greater increase in lean body mass than the casein group (5.0 kilograms versus 0.8 kilogram) and greater fat loss (1.5 kilograms versus 0.2 kilogram). And the group taking whey demonstrated a greater increase in muscle strength.

According to the findings of this study, eating 10 grams of milk proteins by untrained people before and after training combined with strength exercises prompted an increase in the number of satellite muscle cells by 63 percent in two months, which directly affected the regeneration of muscle proteins after training.

Soy Protein Supplements

There are several vegetable-based alternatives for protein supplements. The most popular and most readily available is soy protein. It contains all the essential amino acids in proportions appropriate for the body, which is why the soy protein supplement is usually suggested as a suitable substitute for animal protein. In addition, soy is a source of antioxidants, potassium, zinc, iron, and B vitamins.

Soy protein is among the most digestible plant protein sources (recall the BV and PDCAAS ratings discussed in Chapter 3). However, in comparison to whey protein, the content of leucine and valine belonging to the branched-chain amino acid group is slightly lower. The content of glutamine and arginine is higher, though.

So how does soy protein compare to whey protein? In more than one study assessing soy and whey protein supplementation, no significant differences in muscle mass gain or body composition were found.

Concerns about the use of soy protein stem from the presence of phytosterols in soy (vegetable substances resembling human cholesterol), which

EVIDENCE SUPPORTS TAKING A COMBINATION OF PROTEIN SUPPLEMENTS

It may be helpful to use more than one type of protein supplement at the same time. One study found that taking 20 grams of protein supplements (14 grams whey with casein and 6 grams of branched-chain amino acids) one hour before and after a strength-training workout significantly accelerated the regeneration and development of muscle mass compared to receiving 20 grams of placebo over 10 weeks. Other studies have also confirmed that a combination including casein can promote the most noticeable results. One group of athletes took a combination of whey supplement with casein (48 grams per day) and another took whey, BCAA, and glutamine supplement (48 grams per day). The casein group experienced the greatest increase in lean body mass.

were thought to have a "feminizing" effect on men. However, soy protein does not affect the level of testosterone or sex hormones in men, as confirmed by numerous studies. In a meta-analysis conducted on more than 30 research projects, no relationship was found between the consumption of soybeans and the reduction in the level of male sex hormones.

Pea and Rice Protein

An alternative to soy protein is pea protein. It is slightly less digestible than soy or whey protein, but its undoubted advantage is its protein content. About 25 grams of protein are found in 30 grams of pea protein product, which is the same ratio as in many whey protein products. In a study conducted on a group of 160 men, the effects of pea and whey protein were compared. Men took 25 grams of one of the protein types for 12 weeks and at the same time underwent upper-body strength training. In the two groups, the observed muscle growth was similar.

Another vegetable protein available is rice protein, which contains an insufficient amount of lysine and smaller amounts of branched-chain amino acids compared to whey protein (see Table 8.1). However, in the results of a study comparing the use of rice and whey protein at a dose of 48 grams, no significant differences in post-workout regeneration were noticed, while muscle growth was different (2.5 kilograms in people supplementing with rice protein and 3.2 kilograms for whey protein).

You can also find hemp protein on the market. It contains all the essential amino acids, but its bioavailability is quite low. Hemp protein has other advantages, though: It is rich in dietary fiber, calcium, and zinc and has small amounts of omega-3 fatty acids. However, attention should be paid to the amount of protein in commercially available protein powders. In one 30-gram portion, you will find about 14 grams of protein plus carbohydrates and fats, so it is difficult to call it purely a protein supplement.

TABLE 8.1 **Amino acid profile of rice and soy proteins relative to the standard egg protein**

Amino Acid	Soy Protein (milligrams per 1 gram protein)	Rice Protein Isolate (milligrams per 1 gram protein)	Egg Protein (milligrams per 1 gram protein)
Histidine	19	22	18
Tryptophan	14	14	7
Threonine	38	35	27
Isoleucine	49	41	25
Leucine	82	80	55
Lysine	64	31	51
Methionine	26	28	25
Phenylalanine	92	53	47
Valine	48	58	32

The optimal solution for people who do not want to use soy and whey protein are mixtures of other vegetable proteins. Mixtures of rice and pea proteins, or additionally hemp protein, offer a complete set of amino acids and the availability of protein is greater.

Beta-alanine

Beta-alanine is an amino acid that is a component of carnosine dipeptide, responsible for maintaining the acid-base balance in tissues. In addition, it has antioxidative and chelating effects (it reduces the toxicity of metal ions). Carnosine dipeptide is considered a natural substance with a beneficial effect on the cardiovascular system that inhibits the aging process. Consuming high-carnosine foods, especially from chicken, can inhibit the onset of influenza and cold virus infections.

Carnosine buffers the rise in acidity that comes with increased levels of lactate in the muscles. Carnosine's contribution to reducing muscle fatigue is considered its main role in an athlete's nutrition. Muscle fatigue can be caused by several different factors: One of them is central fatigue, affecting the central nervous system; the second is peripheral fatigue, which consists of a reduction in the muscle's ability to contract by increasing the temperature and acidifying the intracellular environment. This is due to the following:

> Depletion of energy substrates, mainly ATP phosphocreatine and glucose
> Increasing oxidative stress
> Calcium balance disorder, which disturbs the process of muscle contraction
> Accumulation of hydrogen ions (H+) in muscles due to the accumulation of lactate

During a short, intense effort (60–240 seconds long), working muscles derive energy mainly from anaerobic processes (glycolysis). As a result of these transformations, hydrogen ions are formed. An increase in these ions causes a drop in pH, which contributes to the feeling of fatigue. Fortunately, the body has mechanisms that counteract the disturbance of the acid-base balance. One of them is carnosine, formed from an appropriate dose of beta-alanine from food or supplements. Studies show that taking beta-alanine supplements increases the concentration of carnosine in muscle fibers. Thanks to this, the acid-base balance is improved, which can help extend the time an athlete is able to perform.

Positive effects of beta-alanine supplementation have been observed after just four days of use. Although long-term supplementation did not bring any negative health consequences (the maximum test time was 90 days, with daily use), its concentration in the blood and the amount of carnosine in the muscles reached the maximum level after four weeks, so further supplementation does not seem justified.

Athletes using beta-alanine supplementation may feel discomfort in the form of tingling, numbness, or changes in skin temperature. Other side effects appear in the form of itchy skin, most often around the back, abdomen, buttocks, and ears; hot flashes; and shivering. Such effects may occur even if the recommended dose of the supplement is not exceeded. If adverse symptoms occur, the dose should be reduced or the supplement discontinued completely.

Beta-alanine is especially helpful for sprinters, strength sport athletes, or martial artists. This amino acid is easily absorbed by the body, helping muscles take up much more carnosine than they had previously. The recommended dose of beta-alanine is 2.0–6.4 grams per day. Beta-alanine supplementation is also recommended for elderly people undertaking physical activity. Studies show that supplementation of 3.2 grams of beta-alanine daily for 12 weeks significantly improves the exercise capacity of older physically active people.

L-carnitine

L-carnitine is one of the best-known supplements used primarily to reduce body fat. It was first isolated in 1905 from muscles, hence its name (the Latin term for meat is *carn*). An adult needs 15–16 milligrams daily, an amount that can be furnished completely by a typical diet. If necessary, the body is able to synthesize L-carnitine to cover its needs (a 175-pound adult will create 13–38 milligrams per day). Studies show that the amount of L-carnitine delivered daily through food typically ranges from 20 to 200 milligrams, depending on what the individual eats. Diets high in beef can contribute up to 300 milligrams per day. Vegetarian diets can provide as little as 1 milligram per day.

With a proper diet, 75 percent of the daily demand for L-carnitine is covered by food, and the remaining 25 percent is produced by the body. In vegetarians, up to 90 percent of L-carnitine comes from its biosynthesis in the body. L-carnitine is synthesized from two essential amino acids, lysine and methionine, so these acids are important parts of anyone's diet.

The use of fat for energy production can increase by up to 70 percent with the proper amount of L-carnitine. It helps carry coenzyme A (CoA) to the mitochondria, bringing more fat to the energy production process and, as a result, inhibiting the formation of more adipose tissue. As L-carnitine helps fat oxidation, it contributes to the reduction of triglyceride and cholesterol concentrations. Its fat-burning powers help reduce the body's caloric demand and increase tolerance to exercise. Some of the greatest effects of L-carnitine can be seen in people with fat content exceeding 18 percent and 25 percent (in men and women, respectively), especially when they take up a consistent aerobic training program like running or cycling.

L-carnitine has other functions, too. It facilitates the detoxification of the body and is an antioxidant. And it plays an important role in the transformation of carbohydrates. Its abundance in muscles allows you to save glycogen because the body will take more energy from fats, especially valuable in situations of long, aerobic physical activity. This was proven by a group of marathon runners who had very low carnitine levels. The supplementation of L-carnitine at a dose of 2 grams daily for six weeks resulted in the reduction of muscle oxygen consumption, lower heart rates during running, and an increase in the use of fats for energy production.

Research has shown that animal products such as beef and lamb offer some of the highest content, but there's a wide range of L-carnitine concentration in foods: from 4.4 milligrams in 100 grams of chicken to 142 milligrams in 100 grams of beef steak.

The gastrointestinal tract can absorb 50–85 percent of the L-carnitine supplied by food. The remainder is eliminated by the bacteria residing in the large intestine. L-carnitine from supplements is absorbed to a lesser degree: 15–20 percent, and sometimes as little as 5 percent.

Adults are advised to take 250 milligrams to 2 grams of L-carnitine in two to three doses per day. Higher doses (up to 6 grams) can be used by athletes. It is best to take this supplement about one or two hours before training. It can also be taken in the morning after waking up, when its absorption is fastest. Taking one dose at night, about 30 minutes before bedtime, can be beneficial due to its detoxifying and antioxidant action. Carnitine should be taken on an empty stomach and not combined with any meal. According to the latest research, this amino acid gets into the bloodstream within a dozen or so minutes after ingestion. This means that you can eat food 30 minutes after taking it. It is also beneficial to support the slimming effect of L-carnitine with synergistic preparations such as fat burner supplements, conjugated linoleic acid (CLA), hydroxycitric acid, or caffeine. No adverse reactions after the use of oral L-carnitine preparations have been found. Only a few people (a fraction of a percent) had transient reactions on the part of the digestive tract (recurrent nausea, abdominal pain, diarrhea).

It is worth noting, however, that L-carnitine, despite many beneficial properties, will not significantly reduce body fat for everyone; it may not bring about any change in some people, in fact.

Carbohydrate Supplements

Even with a balanced diet, an athlete's supply of carbohydrates through food may need to be boosted by supplements such as sports drinks and gels, but also products designed even more specifically for carbohydrate supply—those found at bodybuilding nutrition stores, for example. Carb supplements can help in glycogen regeneration, which is important for athletes training more than three times per week and especially on back-to-back days.

Taking carbohydrate supplements in a liquid form during training is intended to support the athlete's energy and vitamins and minerals supply.

After training, they ensure quick recovery of energy reserves and the reduction of muscle damage.

Carbohydrate supplements can have a high glycemic index, so their consumption could cause dangerous spikes in insulin. This hormone is helpful, especially in the post-workout phase where it is responsible for the transport of nutrients to muscle cells, but too much of it can cause the deposition of unwanted fat. Therefore, be sure to consume appropriate amounts of carbs before, during, and after training (see Chapter 2 for guidelines on intake).

If you eat a proper meal before a workout, it should provide energy for 60 minutes of intense effort, such as running intervals or a HIIT session. Numerous studies confirm that consuming a carbohydrate drink during a 60-minute workout of moderate intensity will not significantly improve exercise capacity. But keep in mind that every workout, whether it is strength training, running, or general fitness, causes some degree of a drop in glycogen reserves. So, although mid-workout fueling might not be necessary, it is important to take some carbohydrates after the training session.

The need for carbohydrates is completely different during a workout lasting 90 minutes or more. In this case, glycogen resources should be supplemented as early as 45 minutes into training (see "Carbohydrates Before and During Exercise" in Chapter 2). It allows for consistent energy supply without putting too much stress on the digestive system. In this situation, carbohydrates in liquid form will work best, and it's best if they're enriched with vitamins and electrolytes. Energy gels with high carbohydrate content are another option, especially for efforts several hours long like ultramarathons. They are often enriched with caffeine and taurine to stimulate the nervous system. If an athlete uses these types of gels, they should also drink about 200 milliliters of water. Gels aren't always advised during training, but they might be useful during competition. Carb-rich gels are particularly helpful toward the end of a long effort (not at the beginning or before), when not only the muscles, but also the nervous system controlling them are tired.

In strength sports, carbohydrate supplements are quite often used during training. For example, during a gym workout, someone might fuel with a sports drink at the end of weight lifting and then go on to cardio with elevated glycogen so that the muscles are not so depleted. Glycogen being constantly replenished allows for smaller losses during exercise and faster regeneration during recovery.

When someone performs a cardio workout to reduce body fat, the fueling plan looks different. Then, carbs should be delivered only after the workout, and not midway, as in a break between weight lifting and cardio training.

Types of Sugars in Carbohydrate Supplements

Maltodextrins are a group of complex carbohydrates formed as a result of the breakdown of starch. They move quickly through the stomach and do not usually cause intestinal problems. They provide support before, during, and after a physical effort. Besides providing saccharides to be used in glycogen production, maltodextrins accelerate the transport of amino acids necessary for the regeneration and repair of muscle microtears. Maltodextrins have a high glycemic index: at least 80, if not higher.

Dextrose is also used in carbohydrate supplements. It belongs to the group of simple carbohydrates, which means it will be absorbed immediately after consumption. After training, it helps to rebuild muscle glycogen. As a quick-acting fuel source, it can prolong the effort in endurance training.

Vitargo is a patented carbohydrate formula that, according to numerous reports and anecdotal evidence from athletes, works much faster and more efficiently than traditional carbohydrate nutrients. The difference between the original Vitargo and other carbohydrates lies in the molecular weight, which has an effect on the rate of carbohydrate replenishment. Studies have shown that only a carbohydrate with a molecular weight between 500,000 and 700,000 guarantees very fast absorption and replenishment of glycogen. Carbohydrates with other molecular weights are not absorbed as quickly. Regular intake of Vitargo also prevents overtraining, improves the immune system, and reduces the frequency of muscle cramps because of its electrolyte and vitamin supply.

Carbohydrate nutrients sometimes also contain isomaltulose, which interestingly, is composed of two sugars—glucose and fructose—making it quite similar to ordinary white sugar. However, the main difference lies in the type of bonds between these sugars, which gives isomaltulose a low GI (32). Scientific research confirms a much slower rate of energy release from nutrients with isomaltulose, but it also shows the potential side effects of this sugar—primarily gastrointestinal discomfort and abdominal pain.

The combination of glucose or dextrose, maltodextrins, and isomaltulose seems to be an ideal blend in a carbohydrate supplement that can be taken during prolonged physical activity. Each of these sugars releases energy and replenishes glycogen resources at different rates, which is beneficial for the body that needs a steady supply of fuel.

Another carbohydrate nutrient is waxy corn starch. Starch is a carbohydrate consisting of amylopectin and amylose in various proportions. Waxy corn starch is 98 percent amylopectin, and its characteristic feature is the long duration required for it to release energy. It is therefore practical to include it in carbohydrate supplements used before and during a long effort. However, it is not recommended immediately after training, when an athlete needs carbohydrates with a short release time to replenish the body quickly.

Gainers and Combined Protein and Carbohydrate Supplements

After a workout, it's important to replace the carbohydrates that fueled the body. Equally important is the supply of proteins, and more specifically essential amino acids, which will regenerate muscles and contribute to the growth of muscle mass. Supplements containing carbs and protein vary in the proportion of the two nutrients but typically have a predominance of carbs (usually 3 to 1). They are best used immediately after training, but they can also be a meal replacement or a pre-workout meal if you cannot eat a nutritious meal.

These mixes are often used in bodybuilding; "gainers" contain a large amount of protein and carbs. Read the ingredients list of these products and determine the portion size based on what your body needs. If you want a substantial serving of protein but not the carbs that come with it in a gainer, it might be better to consume your protein and carbs separately so that you can control the balance.

Some protein-carbohydrate mixes offer an equal share of both substrates (1 to 1). Many "bulking agents" fall into this category. High-quality proteins provide a steady supply of all essential amino acids, while the mixture of carbohydrates provides fuel and supports the growth of lean body mass. Bulkers are often supplemented with anabolic and anticatabolic amino acids to enhance their effect on the muscles. Bulk supplements, thanks to properly selected food ingredients, can also be a meal replacement, but not more often than once per day.

Meal Replacements

These are supplementary compositions that can completely replace a nutritious meal. Although bulkers or gainers can also replace a meal, meal replacements have a richer mix of wholesome proteins, simple and complex carbohydrates, and polyunsaturated fatty acids. Fiber is often added, too, as well as digestive enzymes that facilitate the digestion of all ingredients and absorption into the body. Some athletes who have regularly occurring gastrointestinal distress use meal replacements. For example, an athlete who can't consume standard meals before training (even far in advance) could use a replacement because it won't cause digestive problems, but it still provides the energy and micronutrients necessary for training.

Probiotics and Prebiotics

The gut contains trillions of bacteria that are helpful and in fact essential for our health. Certain strains of bacteria colonize the digestive tract after entering the body. Eating probiotics—foods that contain more of these beneficial organisms—maintains the health of the bacterial population.

After probiotics are absorbed into the intestine, the microorganisms adhere to its walls, protecting the body from harmful bacteria that can cause infection and illness. Probiotics also support the body in dealing with ailments such as respiratory tract infections, intestinal diseases, weakened immunity, diarrhea, digestive problems, and skin diseases. It is also believed that the consumption of products with probiotic bacteria may be important in the prevention of coronary heart disease. And the latest scientific research has shown that probiotics can reduce damage caused by oxidation, which often accompanies athletic training.

When anyone takes antibiotics for the treatment of a serious infection, the beneficial intestinal microflora can be suppressed for several months or even years. The use of probiotics is therefore indispensable after a regimen of antibiotics. Probiotics can be taken through supplement form like pills or powdered drink mixes, but also in fermented foods such as yogurt, traditional sauerkraut, and kimchi. Thanks to the production of the enzyme beta-galactosidase, bacteria improve the digestion of lactose, which can alleviate gastrointestinal problems related to consuming milk products.

Substances known as prebiotics (as opposed to *pro*biotics) can support healthy bacterial growth in the colon. They are not microorganisms, but rather food (plant-derived fiber) for the beneficial bacteria in the body. As a supplement in the diet, prebiotics can significantly improve one's health and wellbeing. Studies from 2017 indicate that prebiotics may play an important role in the prevention of osteoporosis, obesity, and even colon cancer. Prebiotics can be found in starchy and fibrous foods like whole grains and many vegetables and fruits. Inulin, a type of fiber found in cereals, onions, and bananas, is also a prebiotic.

Pre-workout Supplements

Pre-workout supplements are becoming popular, but they should be taken with caution. The concern lies mainly in the quality of the products. Manufacturers of these supplements ensure their effectiveness in improving efficiency, strength, endurance, and motivation. Many people, including high-performance athletes, consider these supplements to be a golden ticket to the most effective workout they can put forth each day. Unfortunately, quite often this turns out to be problematic and ineffective in the long run.

Pre-workout supplements contain a long list of ingredients, but products vary in what they offer. Many contain substances that affect the central nervous system to stimulate the mind and the perceived energy level so that the athlete can work harder or longer and maintain concentration and resistance to fatigue. Caffeine is therefore a common ingredient. Beta-alanine, mentioned earlier, appears in many compounds because it acts as a blood buffer, increasing the body's adaptation to intense efforts. In pre-workout supplements, you will also find arginine (a precursor of nitric oxide), which causes the expansion of blood vessels, as well as many other stimulants, including Chinese magnolia vine and yerba maté. Other ingredients include creatine, taurine, and antioxidants such as vitamin C or the B-group vitamins. In some, you can also find betaine, found in beets, which can increase strength and endurance.

Generally, pre-workout supplements are permissible unless they contain certain compounds that are banned by governing bodies of sports and anti-doping agencies. Beware long-term use, though: The body can adapt to a given supplement over time, becoming less responsive to the stimulants in particular. As the physical response diminishes, athletes often reach for new, stronger compounds with greater potency, which can cause other side effects: palpitations, excessive sweating, or decreased libido. Pre-workout supplements are particularly dangerous for people with heart disease, hypertension, or nervous-system disorders. Pay close attention if DMAA is listed in the ingredients. A geranium extract, DMAA contains the active substance methylhexanamine, which stimulates the nervous system and causes a thermogenic action. It is dangerous to your health and is a banned substance in sports.

Some pre-workout supplements that are banned by the World Anti-Doping Agency, such as ephedrine and yohimbine, are still available on the market. These types of compounds are very dangerous to your health and even your life.

Nutrition Roundup

Supplements can augment a well-balanced diet of wholesome foods, but they cannot replace it. Depending on your needs, you can choose between supplements that improve your endurance or capacity for training, increase muscle mass or strength, accelerate regeneration of body tissue, or reduce body weight.

Improperly used, especially without a proper diet, supplements can cause adverse effects, so take them with caution and preferably under the supervision of a physician, experienced dietitian, or trainer. Be cautious of information found on the internet or other unofficial sources; in most cases, advice about supplements and doping agents does not come from qualified experts.

Always buy supplements from a safe, trusted, well-known source. In products sold from questionable sources, not all ingredients may be disclosed on the label, or an ingredient listed on the label may not actually be in the product. Research brands and products before making a purchase.

Some supplements contain harmful substances or those that are not permitted by international or national governing bodies of sports. Some products carry "doping-free" or "drug-free" labels, and you can probably trust those a little more, but still give them your due diligence.

CHAPTER 1: POWERING THE ATHLETE

Farias LF Jr, Browne RAV, Frazão DT, et al. Effect of low-volume high-intensity interval exercise and continuous exercise on delayed-onset muscle soreness in untrained healthy males. *J Strength Cond Res.* 2017 Jun 12.

Fogelholm M. Exercise, substrate oxidation and energy balance. *Int J Obesity* 2006;30:1022.

Kenney W, Wilmore J, Costill D. *Physiology of sport and exercise.* 6th ed. Champaign (IL): Human Kinetics; 2015. p. 648

Lazzer S, Tringali G, Caccavale M, et al. Effects of high-intensity interval training on physical capacities and substrate oxidation rate in obese adolescents. *J Endocrinol Invest.* 2017;40(2):217–226.

O'Neill T, Skelton A. Indoor rowing training guide. Nottingham (England): *Concept 2*; 2001. p. 27.

Paoli A, Pacelli F, Bargossi AM, et al. Effects of three distinct protocols of fitness training on body composition, strength and blood lactate. *J Sports Med Phys Fitness.* 2010;50(1):43–51.

CHAPTER 2: CARBOHYDRATES

Atkinson G, Taylor CE, Morgan N, et al. Pre-race dietary carbohydrate intake can independently influence sub-elite marathon running performance. *Int J Sports Med.* 2011;32(8):611–617.

Brand-Miller J, Buyken AE. The glycemic index issue. *Curr Opin Lipidol.* 2012;23(1): 62–67.

Berardi JM, Price TB, Noreen EE, et al. Postexercise muscle glycogen recovery enhanced with a carbohydrate-protein supplement. *Med Sci Sports Exerc.* 2006;38(6):1106–1113.

Burke LM, Cox GR, Culmmings NK, et al. Guidelines for daily carbohydrate intake: do athletes achieve them? *Sports Med.* 2001;31:267–299.

Centeno V, de Barboza GD, Marchionatti A, et al. Molecular mechanisms triggered by low-calcium diets. *Nutr Res Rev.* 2009;22:163–174.

Cermak NM, van Loon LJ. The use of carbohydrates during exercise as an ergogenic aid. *Sports Med.* 2013;43(11):1139–1155.

Chalcarz W, Merkel S, Mikołajczyk A, et al. Spożycie witamin i składników mineralnych w przeddzień meczu, w dzień meczu i po meczu [Consumption of vitamins and minerals on the day before the match, on the match day, and after the match]. *Bromat Chem Toksykol.* 2008;41(3):681–685. Polish.

Christensen DL, Van Hall G, Hambraeus L. Food and macronutrient intake of male adolescent Kalenjin runners in Kenya. *Br J Nutr.* 2002;88:711–717.

Hawley JA, Leckey JJ. Carbohydrate dependence during prolonged, intense endurance exercise. *Sports Med.* 2015;45(Suppl 1):S5–S12.

Huang S, Czech MP. The GLUT4 glucose transporter. *Cell Metab.* 2007;5(4):237–252.

Knuiman P, Hopman MT, Mensink M, et al. Glycogen availability and skeletal muscle adaptations with endurance and resistance exercise. *Nutr Metab (Lond).* 2015;21(12):59.

Lambert CP, Frank LL, Evans WJ. Macronutrient considerations for the sport of bodybuilding. *Sports Med.* 2004;34(5):317–327.

Lis D, Stellingwerff T, Kitic CM, et al. No effects of a short-term gluten-free diet on performance in nonceliac athletes. *Med Sci Sports Exerc.* 2015;47(12):2563–2570.

McCleave EL, Ferguson-Stegall L, Ding Z, et al. A low carbohydrate-protein supplement improves endurance performance in female athletes. *J Strength Cond Res.* 2011;25(4):879–888.

Mikołajczak J, Bator E, Bronowska M, et al. Wartości indeksów i ładunków glikemicznych wybranych płatków zbożowych spożywanych z mlekiem [Values of glycemic indexes and glycemic loads of selected cereal flakes consumed with milk]. *Rocz Państw Zakl Hig.* 2012;63(4):433–440. Polish.

Okazaki K, Goto M, Nose H. Protein and carbohydrate supplementation increases aerobic and thermoregulatory capacities. *J Physiol.* 2009;587:5585–5590.

Panahi S, El Khoury D, Kubant R, et al. Mechanism of action of whole milk and its components on glycemic control in healthy young men. *J Nutr Biochem.* 2014;25(11):1124–1131.

Piehl-Aulin K, Soderlund K, Hultman E. Muscle glycogen resynthesis rate in humans after supplementation of drinks containing carbohydrates with low and high molecular masses. *Eur J Appl Physiol.* 2000;81:346–351.

Raman A, Macdermid PW, Mündel T, et al. The effects of carbohydrate loading 48 hours before a simulated squash match. *Int J Sport Nutr Exerc Metab.* 2014;24(2):157–165.

Wilson PB, Ingraham SJ, Lundstrom C, et al. Dietary tendencies as predictors of marathon time in novice marathoners. *Int J Sport Nutr Exerc Metab.* 2013;23(2):170–177.

CHAPTER 3: PROTEIN

Bonjour JP. Dietary protein: an essential nutrient for bone health. *J Am Coll Nutr.* 2005;24(6):526S–536S.

Campbell B, Kreider RB, Ziegenfuss T, et al. International Society of Sports Nutrition position stand: protein and exercise. *J Int Soc Sports Nutr.* 2007;26(4):8.

Cichosz G, Czeczot H. Kontrowersje wokół białek diety [Controversies around diet proteins]. *Pol Merkur Lek.* 2013;35(210): 397–401. Polish.

Grillenberger M, Neumann CG, Murphy SP, et. al. Intake of micronutrients high in animal-source foods is associated with better growth in rural Kenyan school children. *Brit J Nutr.* 2006;95:379–390.

Helms ER, Zinn C, Rowlands DS, et al. High-protein, low-fat, short-term diet results in less stress and fatigue than moderate-protein moderate-fat diet during weight loss in male weightlifters: a pilot study. *Int J Sport Nutr Exerc Metab.* 2015;25(2):163–170.

Hoffman JR, Falvo MJ. Protein—which is best? *J Sports Sci Med.* 2004;3(3):118–130.

Hulmi JJ, Lockwood CM, Stout JR. Effect of protein/essential amino acids and resistance training on skeletal muscle hypertrophy: a case for whey protein. *Nutr Metab (Lond).* 2010;17(7):51.

Kunachowicz H, Czarnowska-Misztal E, Turlejksa H. Zasady żywienia człowieka [Rules of human nutrition]. Warsaw: *WSiP*; 2007, pp. 23–54. Polish.

Leidy HJ, Clifton PM, Astrup A, et al. The role of protein in weight loss and maintenance. *J Clin Nutr Am.* 2015, pii: ajcn084038.

Massey LK. Dietary animal and plant protein and human bone health: a whole foods approach. *J Nutr.* 2003;133(3):862S–865S.

Moore DR, Robinson MJ, Fry JL, et al. Ingested protein dose response of muscle and albumin protein synthesis after resistance exercise in young men. *Am J Clin Nutr.* 2009;89(1):161–168.

Norton LE, Wilson GJ. Optimal protein intake to maximize muscle protein synthesis: examinations of optimal meal protein intake and frequency for athletes. *Agro Food Industry Hi-Tech.* 2009;20(2):54–57.

Pasiakos SM, McLellan TM, Lieberman HR. The effects of protein supplements on muscle mass, strength, and aerobic and anaerobic power in healthy adults: a systematic review. *Sports Med.* 2015;45(1):111–131.

Rodriguez NR, Di Marco NM, Langley S. American College of Sports Medicine position stand. Nutrition and athletic performance. *Med Sci Sports Exerc.* 2009;41(3):709–731.

Szponara L, Ciok J. Suplementacja a zdrowie człowieka [Supplementation and human health]. Warsaw: *Instytut Żywności i Żywienia*; 2002. p. 48. Polish.

Tarnopolsky MA. Nutritional consideration in the aging athlete. *Clin J Sport Med.* 2008;18(6):531–538.

Thomas DT, Erdman KA, Burke LM. American College of Sports Medicine joint position statement. Nutrition and athletic performance. *Med Sci Sports Exerc.* 2016;48(3):543–568.

Tipton KD. Efficacy and consequences of very-high-protein diets for athletes and exercisers. *Proc Nutr Soc.* 2011;70(2):205–214.

Zimecki M. Artym J. Właściwości terapeutyczne białek i peptydów z siary i mleka [Therapeutic properties of proteins and peptides from colostrum and milk]. *Postępy Hig Med Dośw.* 2005;59:309–323. Polish.

CHAPTER 4: FATS

Cichosz G, Czeczot H. Kontrowersje wokół cholesterolu pokarmowego [Controversies around food cholesterol]. *Pol Merkur Lek.* 2012;33(193):38–42. Polish.

DiNicolantonio JJ, Lucan SC, O'Keefe JH. The evidence for saturated fat and for sugar related to coronary heart disease. *Prog Cardiovasc Dis.* 2016;58(5):464–472.

Lajous M, Bijon A, Fagherazzi G, et al. Egg and cholesterol intake and incident type 2 diabetes among French women. *Br J Nutr.* 2015;114(10):1667–1673.

Lun V, Erdman KA, Reimer RA. Evaluation of nutritional intake in Canadian high-performance athletes. *Clin J Sport Med.* 2009;19(5):405–411.

Oh K, Hu FB, Manson JE, et al. Dietary fat intake and risk of coronary heart disease in women: 20 years of follow-up of the nurses' health study. *Am J Epidemiol.* 2005;161(7):672–679.

Paoli A, Bianco A, Grimaldi KA. The ketogenic diet and sport: a possible marriage? *Exerc Sport Sci Rev.* 2015;43(3):153–162.

Sacks FM, Lichtenstein AH, Wu JHY, et al. Dietary fats and cardiovascular disease: a presidential advisory from the American Heart Association. *Circulation.* 2017;136:e1–e23.

Schick EE. The role of the ketogenic diet in exercise performance. *Medicina Sportiva* 2016;XII(2):2756–2761.

Shin JY, Xun P, Nakamura Y, et al. Egg consumption in relation to risk of cardiovascular disease and diabetes: a systematic review and meta-analysis. *Am J Clin Nutr.* 2013;98(1):146–159.

Strong RC, Hulstein MFE, Meer R. Bovine milk fat components inhibit food-borne pathogens. *Inter. Dairy J.* 2002;12:209–215.

Xu J, Eilat-Adar S, Loria C, et al. Dietary fat intake and risk of coronary heart disease: the Strong Heart Study. *Am J Clin Nutr.* 2006;84(4):894–902.

US Department of Health and Human Services and US Department of Agriculture. 2015–2020 dietary guidelines for Americans. Appendix 7. 8th ed. December 2015. Available at https://health.gov/dietaryguidelines/2015/guidelines/.

Virtanen JK, Mursu J, Tuomainen TP. Egg consumption and risk of incident type 2 diabetes in men: the Kuopio Ischaemic Heart Disease Risk Factor Study. *Am J Clin Nutr*. 2015;101(5):1088–1096.

CHAPTER 5: HYDRATION

American College of Sports Medicine position stand. Nutrition and athletic performance. *Med Sci Sports Exerc*. 2009;41(3):709–731.

Garth AK, Burke LM. What do athletes drink during competitive sporting activities? *Sports Med*. 2013;43(7):539–564.

Maughan RJ. Alcohol and football. *J Sports Sci*. 2006;24(7):741–748.

Maughan RJ. Water and electrolyte loss and replacement in training and competition. In: Maughan RJ, editor. *Sport nutrition: the encyclopaedia of sports medicine*. An IOC Medical Commission publication., Chichester (UK): Wiley-Blackwell; 2014. p. 174–184.

Moore MJ, Werch CE. Sport and physical activity participation and substance use among adolescents. *J Adolesc Health*. 2005;36(6):486–493.

Nuccio RP, Barnes KA, Carter JM, et al. Fluid balance in team sport athletes and the effect of hypohydration on cognitive, technical, and physical performance. *Sports Med*. 2017 Oct;47(10):1951–1982.

Salinero JJ, Lara B, Abian-Vicen J, et al. The use of energy drinks in sport: perceived ergogenicity and side effects in male and female athletes. *Br J Nutr*. 2014;112(9):1494–1502.

Rodriguez NR, DiMarco NM, Langley S. Position of the American Dietetic Association, Dietitians of Canada, and the American College of Sports Medicine: nutrition and athletic performance. *Medscape*. 2010:1–12.

Seifert S, Schaechter J, Hershorin E, et al. Sports drinks and energy drinks for children and adolescents: are they appropriate? *Pediatrics*. 2011;127:1182–1189.

Suzuki K, Hashimoto H, Oh T, et al. The effects of sports drink osmolality on fluid intake and immunoendocrine responses to cycling in hot conditions. *J Nutr Sci Vitaminol*. (Tokyo) 2013;59(3):206–212.

Urso C, Brucculeri S, Caimi G. Hyponatremia and physical exercise. *Clin Ter.* 2012;163(5):e349–e356.

Verster JC, Koenig J. Caffeine intake and its sources: a review of national representative studies. *Crit Rev Food Sci Nutr.* 2017 Feb;16:1–10.

Warzak WJ, Evans S, Floress MT, et al. Caffeine consumption in young children. *J Pediatr.* 2011;158(3):508–509.

Zhang Y, Coca A, Casa DJ, et al. Caffeine and diuresis during rest and exercise: a meta-analysis. *J Sci Med Sport.* 2015;18(5):569–574.

CHAPTER 6: SAMPLE MEAL PLANS

Burke L, Hawley J, Wong S, et al. Carbohydrates for training and competition. *J Sports Sci.* 2011;29 (Suppl):17–27.

Campbell B, Kreider RB, Ziegenfuss T, et al. International Society of Sports Nutrition position stand: protein and exercise. *J Int Soc Sports Nutr.* 2007;26(4):8.

Hargreaves M, Hawley JA, Jeukendrup A. Preexercise carbohydrate and fat ingestion: effects on metabolism and performance. *J Sports Sci.* 2004;22(1):31–38.

Institute of Medicine. *Dietary reference intakes for energy, carbohydrate, fiber, fat, fatty acids, cholesterol, protein, and amino acids.* Washington (DC): National Academies Press; 2005.

Jeukendrup A. Nutrition for endurance sports: marathon, triathlon, and road cycling. *J Sports Sci.* 2011;29:91–99.

Kasprzak Z, Pilaczynska-Szczesniak L, Czubaszewski L. Strategie żywieniowe w wysiłkach wytrzymałościowych [Nutritional strategies in endurance efforts]. *Studia i Materiały Centrum Edukacji Przyrodniczo-Leśnej* 2013;15(34):104–110. Polish.

Lun V, Erdman KA, Reimer RA. Evaluation of nutritional intake in Canadian high-performance athletes. *Clin J Sport Med.* 2009;19(5):405–411.

Maughan R, Burke L. Żywienie a zdolność do wysiłku [Nutrition and the ability to exercise]. Kraków: *Medicina Sportiva*; 2000. Polish

Mizera K, Mizera J. Dieta piłkarska. Nawadnianie [Soccer diets. Hydration]. *Sport Wyczynowy.* 2012;3:71–83.

Mizera K, Mizera J. Żywienie w sportach wytrzymałościowych uprawianych na rekreacyjnym i wyczynowym poziomie [Nutrition in endurance sports practiced at recreational and high-performance levels]. *Zarządzanie i Edukacja* 2012;85:64–81. Polish.

Mizera K, Pilis W. Znaczenie żywienia w sportach siłowych w różnych fazach ontogenezy człowieka [The importance of nutrition in strength sports in various phases of human ontogeny]. *Med Sportiva Pract.* 2008;9(4):73–84. Polish.

Rapaport B. Metabolic factors limiting performance in marathon runners. *PLoS Comput Biol.* 2010;6(10):1–12.

Rodriguez NR, DiMarco NM, Langley S, et al. Position of the American Dietetic Association, Dietitians of Canada, and the American College of Sports Medicine: nutrition and athletic performance. *J Am Diet Assoc.* 2009;109(3):509–527.

Thomas DT, Erdman KA, Burke LM. American College of Sports Medicine Joint Position Statement. Nutrition and athletic performance. *Med Sci Sports Exerc.* 2016;48(3):543–568.

CHAPTER 8: NUTRITIONAL SUPPLEMENTS

Artioli GG, Gualano B, Smith A, et al. Role of beta-alanine supplementation on muscle carnosine and exercise performance. *Med Sci Sports Exerc.* 2010;42(6):1162–1173.

Babizhayev MA, Deyev AI. Management of the virulent influenza virus infection by oral formulation of nonhydrolized carnosine and isopeptide of carnosine attenuating proinflammatory cytokine-induced nitric oxide production. *Am J Ther.* 2012;19(1):e25–e47.

Bassit RA, Pinheiro CH, Vitzel KF, et al. Effect of short-term creatine supplementation on markers of skeletal muscle damage after strenuous contractile activity. *Eur J Appl Physiol.* 2010;108(5):945–955.

Bemben MG, Witten MS, Carter JM, et al. The effects of supplementation with creatine and protein on muscle strength following a traditional resistance training program in middle-aged and older men. *J Nutr Health Aging.* 2010; 14(2):155–159.

Burd NA, Yang Y, Moore DR, et al. Greater stimulation of myofibrillar protein synthesis with ingestion of whey protein isolate v. micellar casein at rest and after resistance exercise in elderly men. *Br J Nutr*. 2012;108(6):958–962.

Campbell B, Roberts M, Kerksick C, et al. Pharmacokinetics, safety, and effects on exercise performance of L-arginine alpha-ketoglutarate in trained adult men. *Nutrition*. 2006;22(9):872–881.

Derave W, Everaert I, Beeckman S, et al. Muscle carnosine metabolism and beta-alanine supplementation in relation to exercise and training. *Sports Med*. 2010;40(3):247–263.

Devries MC, Phillips SM. Supplemental protein in support of muscle mass and health: advantage whey. *J Food Sci*. 2015;80 (Suppl 1):A8–A15.

Filippin LI, Moreira AJ, Marroni NP, et al. Nitric oxide and repair of skeletal muscle injury. *Nitric Oxide*. 2009;21(3–4):157–163.

Hickner RC, Dyck DJ, Sklar J, et al. Effect of 28 days of creatine ingestion on muscle metabolism and performance of a simulated cycling road race. *J Int Soc Sports Nutr*. 2010;7:26.

Hill D, Sugrue I, Arendt E, et al. Recent advances in microbial fermentation for dairy and health. *F1000Res*. 2017 May 26;6:751.

House JD, Neufeld J, Leson G. Evaluating the quality of protein from hemp seed (Cannabis sativa L.) products through the use of the protein digestibility-corrected amino acid score method. *J Agric Food Chem*. 2010;58(22):11801–11807.

Huang WC, Chang YC, Chen YM, et al. Whey protein improves marathon-induced injury and exercise performance in elite track runners. *Int J Med Sci*. 2017;14(7):648–654.

Jäger R, Kerksick CM, Campbell BI, et al. International society of sports nutrition position stand: protein and exercise. *J Int Soc Sports Nutr*. 2017;14:20.

Kim DH, Kim SH, Jeong WS, et al. Effect of BCAA intake during endurance exercises on fatigue substances, muscle damage substances, and energy metabolism substances. *J Exerc Nutrition Biochem*. 2013;17(4):169–180.

Kerksick CM, Rasmussen CJ, Lancaster SL, et al. The effects of protein and amino acid supplementation on performance and training adaptations during ten weeks of resistance training. *J Strength Cond Res*. 2006;20(3):643–653.

Koo GH, Woo J, Kang S, et al. Effects of supplementation with BCAA and L-glutamine on blood fatigue factors and cytokines in juvenile athletes submitted to maximal intensity rowing performance. *J Phys Ther Sci.* 2014;26(8):1241–1246.

Law YL, Ong WS, GillianYap TL, et al. Effects of two and five days of creatine loading on muscular strength and anaerobic power in trained athletes. *J Strength Cond Res.* 2009;23(3):906–914.

Legault Z, Bagnall N, Kimmerly DS. The influence of oral L-glutamine supplementation on muscle strength recovery and soreness following unilateral knee extension eccentric exercise. *Int J Sport Nutr Exerc Metab.* 2015;25(5):417–426.

Mizera K, Mizera J. Wpływ wybranych suplementów diety na sportowców dyscyplin siłowych trenujących wyczynowo i rekreacyjnie [Impact of selected dietary supplements on athletes of power disciplines training in high-performance and recreational activities]. *Zesz Nauk Almamer.* 2015;1(74):57–71. Polish.

Sharp CP, Pearson DR. Amino acid supplements and recovery from high-intensity resistance training. *J Strength Cond Res.* 2010;24(4):1125–1130.

Song QH, Xu RM, Zhang QH, et al. Glutamine supplementation and immune function during heavy load training. *Int J Clin Pharmacol Ther.* 2015;53(5):372–376.

Tang JE, Lysecki PJ, Manolakos JJ, et al. Bolus arginine supplementation affects neither muscle blood flow nor muscle protein synthesis in young men at rest or after resistance exercise. *J Nutr.* 2011;141(2):195–200.

Tobias G, Benatti FB, de Salles Painelli V, et al. Additive effects of beta-alanine and sodium bicarbonate on upper-body intermittent performance. *Amino Acids.* 2013;45(2):309–317.

van Loon LJ, Gibala MJ. Dietary protein to support muscle hypertrophy. *Nestle Nutr Inst Workshop Ser.* 2011;69:79–89, discussion 89–95.

Wang Y, Wu Y, Wang Y, et al. Antioxidant properties of probiotic bacteria. *Nutrients.* 2017;9(5):521.

Yuan J, Jiang B, Li K, et al. Beneficial effects of protein hydrolysates in exercise and sports nutrition. *J Biol Regul Homeost Agents.* 2017;31(1):183–188.

INDEX

ABOUT THE AUTHORS

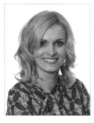

Justyna Mizera, MA, is a sports nutritionist who has developed more than one thousand diets for various sports. She has worked with 30 world-championship medalists and Olympians, but also everyday athletes and children. She has competed in fitness competitions and two half-marathons. The author of numerous scientific and popular science articles, Justyna serves as a nutrition expert for some of the largest television stations in Poland. She was also a dietitian in the television program *Run Back the Clock*. She teaches classes in the field of dietetics.

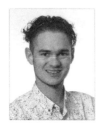

Krzysztof Mizera, PhD, is a sports physiologist and personal trainer. He works with leading athletes and amateurs in the fields of training, weight loss, motor skill improvement, performance testing, and nutrition. Since 2008, Krzysztof has served as a lecturer at various universities. A contributor to numerous scientific projects and conferences, his doctoral thesis examined nutrition and training in strength sports. He is the author of more than 120 publications and the bestseller *Running Is Simple*, and he founded the Olimpiakos Centre. He has run five half-marathons.